I0441012

A Bamboo Grove for the Soul

A Storybook of Spiritual Resources for Caregivers

Tom Becraft, MA, BCC
Board Certified Chaplain

What Readers are Saying:

"Becraft shares stories that remind us of the awe and mystery of our human journey. He pushes us to look deeply at difficult aspects of that journey, and does so with a grace and practicality inspiring to anyone who is in the caregiver role." – Susan Frampton, PhD, President, Planetree, Derby, CT

"A beautiful introduction to caregiving and how chaplains sustain their faith and vitality through the darkness of human experience. Few are as qualified to speak to such challenges. Fewer still are able to write so eloquently about them." – Tom Adams, MDiv, LMFT, Director of Chaplain Services, Tri-Cities Chaplaincy, Kennewick, WA

"Becraft made me laugh and cry with his stories and then provided amazing tools. He gives of himself to create a very readable resource that can be easily utilized by caregivers." – Meg Fallows, MBA, Volunteer Coordinator, Kadlec Regional Medical Center, Richland, WA

"*A Bamboo Grove for the Soul* is a profound exploration of concepts, experiences and emotions, yet it remains easily readable, even by persons unacquainted with theological or psychological theories. Sprinkled with intercultural and personal illustrations, it opens windows on the world while exploring the depths of the soul. Sensitive to interfaith issues, Becraft uses a variety of approaches to accomplish his purpose: poignant stories, helpful descriptive and didactic information, biographical sketches and reflections. These model healing ministry and restore the emotions of stressed caregivers. He gives a gripping portrayal of chaplaincy at its most intense and best." – Darold Bigger, PhD, MDiv, MSW, Rear Admiral, Chief of Chaplains, United States Naval Reserve, Retired; Professor of Religion and Social Work, Walla Walla University, Walla Walla, WA

"WOW! WOW! WOW! WOW! WOW! My husband and I are sitting here being blessed as we glean 'gems' from the depths of your life experience. Thank you for sharing, caring and uplifting our hearts and souls into the vast presence of God." – Lorraine Nichols, RN, Patient Advocate, Surprise, AZ

It's for you!

The Readers

A Bamboo Grove for the Soul was written for caregivers who want to care more competently and compassionately, who wonder if their caregiving matters. It is especially for those who want deeper experiences with the Sacred alongside the hurting, grieving, sick, and dying. Among those who will be energized by this book are:

- Clinicians such as hospital chaplains, family counselors, social workers, nurses, and doctors.
- Community leaders such as clergy and life educators.
- Highly stressed people who are seeking coping resources.

The Breeze Beneath my Wings

A Bamboo Grove for the Soul is dedicated with inexpressible gratitude:

- First to my beloved wife, Bonnie Oneonta-Becraft, LMFT, BCC, a fellow chaplain who lovingly shows what it means to live with integrity and commitment day after day in a journey of ceaseless pain and quiet faith.
- Secondly to my chaplain colleagues at Tri-Cities Chaplaincy who share the wisdom of their experience year after year with presence, passion and purpose.
- And finally to all who yearn for wholeness of body, mind and spirit.

A Bamboo Grove for the Soul

Printed in the United States of America

ISBN-13: 978-1481016551

Learn more at: www.Tom-Becraft.com

CONFESSION TIME

Yes, you might think you recognize yourself or a loved one somewhere in *A Bamboo Grove for the Soul*. If so, I am glad because my intent is to invite you into a story that feels like your own *even when it is not*.

I confess. Though all vignettes are true, I've falsified details to mask the identity of patients, families, and their caregivers. I've taken great care to protect information that could be attributed to any specific individual. In most cases, names are not true. Times are not true. Room numbers are not true. Diseases and diagnoses are changed. Even gender and culture have been manipulated. Based on these changes, one might call this a book of fiction. At the same time, the fundamental mood and dialog of each situation remains true to what I encountered. If you think I am writing expressly about you, please know that it is not so. At the same time, I want your imagination to claim a connection.

While providing resources, my goal has been to capture and portray the essence of spiritual caregiving by sharing when, where, and how the Sacred appears. As the Holy One appears to you in this book, you will know who you are.

To the extent that you claim a piece of any story as an expression of your own journey, I claim gratitude for the privilege of walking alongside and learning from you and those like you.

Wishing you peace,

Tom Becraft, BCC

TABLE OF CONTENTS

Introduction

WELCOME
TO THE BAMBOO GROVE

The tsunami and earthquake-ravaged landscape of Japan shook me to my core. Hour after hour I awaited gut-wrenching news from towns and cities across the Pacific where former colleagues, students and friends might be dead. Each day, week after week, I watched discouraging news and awaited word of survivors. Imagine my joy when I learned that my friends are alive!

The islands of Japan are dear to my heart, holding many precious memories. Forty years ago I spent ten hours a day in Tokyo striving to master the Japanese language. It was a tough two years leading to several wonderful and challenging decades away from my cultural roots. My efforts to wrap myself around strange sounds and new ways of being often felt infantile and futile. The convolutions of my tongue were frequently matched by the twists and turns of my emotions. Every day shook the equilibrium of my soul.

I saw things I'd never known before. Scaffolding made with bamboo, rising 10 stories high. Men with split-toed boots clambering up and down. As I examined and experienced the unfamiliar, I heard a cacophony of noises whirling like barnstorming gnats around my ears. How does one make sense of it all?

According to ancient Japanese wisdom, when an earthquake strikes, one should immediately retreat into a bamboo thicket. Why? It is not simply that bamboo will flex without breaking, though that is true. It is not simply that a bamboo grove provides a windbreak in gale force winds, though that is also true. It is really about what is out of sight. It is about the root system. When seismic activity rocks the landscape, cracks go *around* the bamboo sanctuary rather than through it. Tuberous roots with tendrils of steel-like strength form a haven for the shaken.

Finally, when the earth stops moving and all around is desolate, there is one more benefit in a bamboo grove. Breakfast, lunch, and supper are at one's fingertips. One can eat the roots, and there will be more the next day. There is safety, strength and sustenance. Therefore, we seek the bamboo grove.

ENGAGING THE MYSTERY

Solomon, king and sage of the Israelites, wrote that God "has planted eternity in the human heart" (Ecclesiastes 3:11, *NLT*), providing a capacity to grow in awareness of all that pertains to life. He observed that our quest brings disappointment and brokenness. Yet, beyond life's pain and despair there is hope. He notes that in the thin place between sickness and wellness, at the final juncture of life and death, we encounter an all-knowing One who willingly companions with us through a mysterious portal to newness. From that vantage point, we see both our past and hints of what is over the horizon. Our DNA looks for a bamboo sanctuary where one may transcend destructive forces.

Jesus, a wisely perceptive rabbi, once said, "Look at the birds of the air, that they do not sow, neither do they reap, nor gather into barns, and yet your heavenly Father feeds them. Are you not worth much more than they?" (Matthew 6:26, *HCSB*). Consider a small brown-speckled bird that winters in Hawaii and summers in Alaska. When spring comes, the adult male and female *Kolea* (Pacific Golden Plover - *Pluvialis fulva*) fly 3,000 miles across the Pacific to the Alaskan tundra where they soon lay a cluster of eggs. After their babies hatch, the new parents return to Hawaii, leaving their fledglings behind. Soon temperatures drop, chilling all that lives. How can the little ones survive? Mysteriously each year the infants escape the devastating winter by flying over the wide ocean on a super skinny trajectory unescorted to a place where they've never been. It is a thin line, a narrow path toward Paradise. These simple birds ultimately gain rest by attending to an inner voice, an invisible compass. Is humankind different?

In our humanity, we often lean into turbulence and pain on the wings of prayer. Yet, in such moments our prayers may feel like fragile feathers in a turbulent jet stream. Strength is elusive. As we strive to voice our needs, our words fail us and all that is left are tears. In those moments our tears become a silent, non-verbal prayer to the Divine to energize us. As precious as blood, our tears wordlessly cry out to the Transcendent One to be seen and acknowledged.

Long ago a grief-filled king cried out to his God, "You keep track of all my sorrows. You have captured all my tears in your bottle" (Psalm 56:8, *NLT*). Picture God holding, not a tissue box, but a giant jar, inviting us to spill ourselves into his hands. Imagine God with his head leaning over the container. The Holy One's tears fall and mingle with ours. In this picture, prayer is about being in community with the Sacred and with one another. It is about finding companionship in a cleansing, healing place. It is about reclaiming faith, hope and love in what might appear at first to be a pool of despair. This is because a Mighty One holds the vessel.

God is present. Every day. Always. Never is a prayer lifted heavenward without the Holy One reaching out in compassion to touch the wounded spirit of the broken-hearted. Even before we articulate the yearnings of our hearts, heavenly grace descends, nudging us toward healing. As our hearts and hands open toward heaven, the muscular arms of God reach out to enfold us, bringing us rest and peace. In those faithful hands is wellness.

WEAVING THE TAPESTRY

Through the years, I have spent countless days alongside patients in that unavoidable gossamer space between mortality and immortality, between this life and whatever comes after. Disease and trauma are very real. I have seen the painful impact of cancer, heart disease and other illnesses. I've also seen people transfigured with joy as they've expired. Each occasion feels somehow holy and compels me to examine my faith.

When a cure is not possible, can we yet anticipate another kind of healing – one that is beyond all treatment plans? Indeed, I believe:

- That both individuals and institutions have a core need for attentiveness toward soul and spirit.
- That pain is a part of both personal and organizational development.
- That such pain can be transformed even as it changes us.
- That wellness within is ultimately more powerful than a bodily cure.
- That the Holy One is breathing transcendent healing toward us at every moment.

Caregivers and patients alike know that hospitals are places where breathing is often labored and rest is elusive. The distance between wellness and brokenness is razor thin and sharp. For patients and their families, an illness is a scalpel splitting the veil between what has been and what might be. During such times, thoughts and emotions do not ask permission; they come unbidden, stirring a yearning for insight into meaning and purpose, and a desire that there be more to life than another blood draw, another tasteless intravenous "meal", or another choice between a snake and a serpent.

Within the context of life and death, this storybook offers to you vignettes of grace and a sampling of prayers, blessings and rituals in three dimensions:

- Personal – private expressions of faith, hope and love.
- Institutional – invocations of divine blessing upon people and places.
- Integrative – a merging of transcendent values in self-paced retreats for individuals within healthcare institutions.

This book is both storybook and handbook. Every story, prayer, blessing and ritual is part of a tapestry that comes from life. All stories are drawn from real situations, but details have been altered to protect confidentiality. The prayers and rituals form a picture of people stretched and framed by life's circumstances. Spread out or wrapped up tightly, the fabric breathes. In and out, every thread dances in community whether colorful, tight, loose, somber or happy. On life's loom, praying and breathing are the warp and weft, intersecting in an ongoing dance of creativity. As elements of life, they are intimate, instinctual and energizing.

It is not happenstance that prayer and breath are metaphorically linked around the world. By breathing we live, and by praying we seek more of life. Whether consciously or not, our bodies and hearts turn outward to receive all that is possible. We innately open ourselves to take in that which cannot always be contained in vessels of flesh. We seek the Sacred beyond ourselves. Thus, throughout *A Bamboo Grove for the Soul*, I will give special attention to how God breathes life into us.

The first portion of *A Bamboo Grove for the Soul* seeks answers to the question, Where is God in this? Indeed, how God reveals the Holy Self in chaotic times and places is intimately surprising and profoundly transformative. When God's face appears to us in certain ways, our personal priorities shift both in how we pray and how we care for others and ourselves. In this section we look to the Creator as our greatest resource for healing human brokenness. The section concludes with "De-stressing in Seven Breaths."

The second section is about community and the soul of an institution. As care providers, we sometimes inquire of individuals, "With all that is happening for you now, how are you within?" This same question may be rephrased for institutions, "What works and what doesn't?" *A Bamboo Grove for the Soul* looks at how individuals interact with one another to build relationships. The Sacred's gossamer beauty is here in people and also in a collection of prayers, blessings and rituals offered at gatherings of people as conveyers of hope.

The third section examines how an individual's passions, skill-set, and sense of divine calling may converge to create teams of spiritual caregivers. This is a practical section that shows how the Holy One equips for service. It is particularly relevant for anyone contemplating a career as a professional chaplain. In this section, I relate some of my own experiences while transitioning into healthcare ministries. Above all, you will encounter the Sacred One as an integrative presence choreographing life in profound movements of grace.

The fourth section introduces a unique way to create non-threatening, soul-renewing experiences in such places as chapels. The creation of contemplative, self-paced retreats changes people one person at a time without sermonizing. Included are suggestions for rituals and prayers that pertain to body-mind-spirit wellness. Each of the sample

5

scripts may be experienced within the pages of this book or developed as part of a chapel's or church's décor to be received as part of a journey of personal integration and inner healing. You have permission to replicate or modify these copyrighted scripts for non-commercial personal and institutional settings. Please include a credit line such as: "Utilized and/or modified with permission by Tom Becraft, author of *A Bamboo Grove for the Soul*, copyright 2014."

The fifth and final section transports readers beyond the world of loss and grief into flowering groves of grace. It is about anticipatory joy.

A Bamboo Grove for the Soul is not a one-size-fits-all prayer book or storybook. In fact, it may not fit some at all. My intent is to provide a landing strip and flying mechanism for readers to navigate in and out of emotional and spiritual pain. Take the tapestry presented here and turn it into a flying carpet, modifying it with your own turbojets. As you reflect on the content, experiences and expressions of spirituality contained here, where does your own heart take you? What would you take out, what would you add? As you live and breathe, I pray that my weaving of divine grace will inspire and elevate you toward higher intimacy with the Most Holy. Soar! And wherever you eventually land, may your touchdown be in a soul-sustaining bamboo grove!

Chapter 1

FINDING
WHAT MATTERS MOST

A gentle, persistent tug on my pant leg grabbed my attention, and I looked downward into the brown-eyed face of Jeremy, a four-year-old boy. A somber smile framed his words. "It's my turn now..."

My own "turn" had begun an hour earlier when I received an urgent phone call from a hospice nurse. "I need a priest here," she said. "Our patient is actively dying." As a healthcare chaplain, one of my roles is to facilitate the honoring of patient's needs and wishes regarding spiritual care. So, I, a Protestant minister, made some quick calls, reaching out to locate a Catholic priest who might come immediately to the patient's home to give "an anointing for the sick." At last, I connected with a parish secretary who informed me that she would send a priest "as soon as possible."

With these assurances, I pondered my next move, and decided to hasten to the patient's home, hoping that my presence might somehow be helpful to them if a priest was not able to make it there in time.

I was greeted at the entrance by one of the patient's ten children, a daughter who tearfully said, "The priest just left. He got here! Thank you!" She then added, "Mom is still breathing. Won't you please come in?" As I stepped across the threshold, I heard her say. "Mom's back in the bedroom. We would like it if you also would come and pray with us."

So, in her wake, I swam through an assemblage of well-wishers, through a living room, through a kitchen and around a tight corner into a spacious bedroom crowded with a large group of children, grandchildren and great-grandchildren. A wizened, white-haired woman lay ensconced on a hospital bed, eyes closed, and breathing with the sporadic, familiar sounds of escaping life. I knew her death would come soon, within the next few days, if not sooner.

Introductions were made. At each turning, I saw faces etched with grief. In the following moments as I stood alongside the patient, I elicited stories from individuals around the room about Maria, the tribal chieftain. The stories unfurled like banners of love in breezes of grace. Sacred air, holy ground – that is what I felt.

Time seemed to tiptoe in surreal increments as Maria's life was sketched with multiple terms of endearment and lengthy embellishments. Then slowly, the voices paused like a drying fountain pen seeking inspiration, searching for the remainder of the story. In their silence they looked at me as if to ask, what next? Thinking of the daughter's earlier request that I pray with them, I asked, "Would it be helpful now to have a little prayer together?"

Spontaneously the clan encircled the bed, pressing tightly together shoulder-to-shoulder, clasping hands with their heads bowed. "Dear Lord," I prayed, "We believe that you see and know the needs and desires of our hearts today. So, hear our prayer now as we release Maria into your loving, gentle hands, trusting that you will hold her close to your heart and affirm to her your love, power, and presence. We ask that you give to her freedom and rest from the struggles of this life. I also ask that you comfort each of her children, grandchildren, great-grandchildren and all her friends in the coming hours and days with your tender touch. Above all else, empower this family with hope. We give you our thanks. Amen."

As the family released their hands and began tearfully moving away from the bed, I suddenly felt a tug on my pant leg, and felt little fingers reaching into my left hand. "Please, Pastor. It is my turn now. I wanna pway," he lisped.

Moving aside, I created room for little Jeremy to stand next to his great-grandma. With the pastoral authority of a seasoned minister, he asked his aunties, uncles and all the greats as well, to once again hold hands. Stretching himself to his full height, he extended his arms over the side of the bed and clasped his grandma's face tenderly between his palms, and then prayed. "Dear Jesus, Gwandma is yours. We love her too. But, she is yours! We give her to you...Amen."

The family stepped back, talking, crying, and laughing in little groups. Jeremy observed them silently for a moment, and then spoke again. "That was good! Let's do it again!" Once more he exhorted them to gather around the bed and hold hands. A second time he prayed, this time with more eloquence and confidence. "Pwease, God, we *all* love Gwandma. We'll miss her. But, it's time now for you to have her. You can have her now."

Once again, silence shouted with pregnant hope and tears as aunties and uncles, cousins and others stepped away from the crowded bedside, clustering in conversation. Jeremy went from group to group. "Don't cwy...Gwandma's okay. She is goin' to a bettah pwace..."

BALANCING PREPAREDNESS AND OPENNESS

Comfort to grieving people indeed comes in big and little ways. And that which is little is so often more. Finding the "right" words for prayer is full of mystery. Yet we know that meaningful and helpful prayers come at an intersection of intentionality and spontaneity. We strive in our spiritual caregiving to find the balance between preparedness and openness toward the unfolding story.

Often our primary task is to stand ready for whatever unfolds. Ian Thomas, a Scottish clergyman, once described this readiness as "restful availability." (W. Ian Thomas, *The Saving Life of Christ,* Zondervan). Restful availability is a mindset and heart-orientation that listens with sensitivity to whatever is in the shadows, in those places of silence. Sometimes our compulsion to help or "fix" something may get in the way of truly hearing. When we do not listen to people's stories and instead automatically focus on saying a prayer or reading a scripture, we risk lopping off people's ears so that they might not hear either prayer or scripture.

Praying effectively means attending first to the story. Indicators of the story may be tears, anger, irritability, or deflective humor. What are the themes that emerge as we hear what brings joy to a person? In the identification of themes we find what brings meaning and purpose. It is often in shadowy places of the human journey that we most clearly see and hear the Sacred One's presence.

When a retired utility pole climber speaks of his hobby of collecting and repairing old "plug 'n pull" switchboards, is there an underlying message about relational pain and the connections that matter most? When a patient rhapsodizes about hours spent fishing for sturgeon, is there something in his story that informs regarding internal battles and victories?

As caregivers, we are called upon to provide a deep kind of listening. By attending to metaphors and sensory indicators, we may find clues to areas of soul pain that may be impeding a therapeutic process. When people are in crisis, we are called to deal more with the language of life than the language of faith, to respond to situations rather than to interpret faith traditions, to find discernment rather than to articulate a specific belief system, to listen for body-wrenching soul pain that is often framed in colorful language.

A man cries, "Sh**!" and then apologizes. If we pay attention and do not condemn we will discover that street language and Biblical language are sometimes quite close. The prophet Isaiah described humankind swimming with cunning hands in barnyard soup (Isaiah 25:11, *NIV*). Later, Jesus, the Lord of the Christian faith, gave Satan a graphic title. He called him, "Beelzebub," Lord of Flies, identifying him as the manure-inhabiting, crap-generating source of human misery. Truly, colorful language may hold important messages. When life is crappy, it is important to find big shovels. Sensitivity helps us find the stench. Prayer becomes the bucket on the tractor of faith that clears the road ahead.

Somewhere in his life Rudy missed the class on anger management. Since being admitted to the hospital, his fists often flew like angry wasps at every caregiver. He rudely spewed verbal venom at doctors and nurses. His family likewise was not immune from his wrath. They said Rudy's tirades were lifelong behaviors. And they did not want him to come home. "We are afraid," they said. "He's always abusive. We never feel safe. We've had enough!"

Finally the staff put Rudy in restraints, tying his wrists to his bedrails. And then they and the family called for a chaplain. After conferencing with family members, I entered alongside the doctor, several nurses and a discharge planner.

One by one the team articulated to Rudy the likely consequences of his behavior, especially of his desire to leave the hospital AMA – "against medical advice." He was told that going home and being abusive there might result in police interventions, and that he would probably die from unresolved medical problems, perhaps in jail if he continued to threaten his family.

He screamed, "I don't care! I don't care if they lock me up. I don't want to be here!" Rudy never shut up, relentlessly directing a stream of profanities and vulgarities to each person. Doctors and nurses stayed calm, focused and firmly polite. Then it was my turn. I introduced myself. "I'm Tom, a hospital chaplain."

Like a puss-filled boil touched by a sharp-tipped scalpel, Rudy exploded again, "Chaplain? You are the BIGGEST m***** f***** of everyone!" Hatred filled his eyes as he sought my reaction.

Instantly my mind flashed to childhood parental warnings about "gutter talk" and bars of soap. But, something inside me kicked in: *Meet people where they are.* A surreal calmness filled me as I quickly sent a "flare prayer" upward for divine wisdom. Quietly, respectfully and firmly, I spoke to Rudy. "I need you to know that I am the 'm***** f*****' who wants to honor and respect your wishes. I am here to support your desires. Are you okay with that?"

Instantly, the room shifted. A shocked Rudy became suddenly quiet, or at least a *little* quieter than he had been. He began to listen. As a team, we then told him what we would do to support his demands. We would put him in a wheel chair, take him to the hospital entrance where he could call whomever he wished to come and take him to a hotel where he could sort out any further decisions. He affirmed that this is what he wanted and that he was willing to accept all risks. Thus, he was soon on his way as I mentally cleansed my mouth out with soap.

"Where is God in this?" is the underlying question as we listen and look for ways to move forward in the midst of chaos. This question is fundamentally different from the questions, "What is needed?" and "How can I fix this?" In our approach to needy, hurting, angry persons, we walk a fine line between throwing ourselves at resolving a problem and allowing the Sacred to infuse the situation with grace that meets people in their language and their pain.

11

Scripture indicates that the early downfall and desert experience of Moses began when he looked "this way and that way" prior to killing a murderous taskmaster (Exodus 2:12 *NIV*). The need for fixing was real, but Moses' solution was not helpful. He certainly did not help himself or his cause. Moses looked every direction except upward, and in so doing removed himself from effective service for four decades. From him we learn that skewed, well-intentioned priorities can cause harm both to caregiver and patient.

Therefore, "Where is God in this?" is a question not only for care recipients, but also one that we ask ourselves. Our prayers are often need-driven. Indeed, circumstances may be so emotionally compelling that we leap to rescue or be rescued before harkening to the Ultimate Editor of our lives. Seeking the Sacred in each encounter is our first priority. Fixing is not. As we seek to see and hear the movements of the Divine One in every person, God appears with indicators of how the slithering serpents of anxiety, fear, and anger might be vanquished. Our upward and inward pause holds space for the Holy One to direct the resolution of pain.

Discovering Strength
Through Vulnerability

Significantly, it was only when Moses turned aside from his sheep-oriented frustrations toward the mystery of a forever-burning bush that the Shepherd of Human Hearts appeared and equipped him with the essentials of leadership. He found resolution for the quandaries of his sheep-ministry when he paused to truly look and hear.

God identified to Moses the basis of caregiver authority. The first message of God to this ancient emancipator was, "Take off your sandals, for you are standing on holy ground" (Exodus 3:5, *NLT*). As care providers we may hear the voice from within the mystery as an invitation to walk with vulnerability. It is an invitation to feel, sense and heed what lies underneath. Desert soil is often rough, rock-strewn, cactus-infested and brutal upon bare feet. Not such a fun place to walk with unclad skin! Yet it is holy ground! Shards of brokenness, including our own, awaken us to what is really important. Like Moses, caregivers are called first and foremost to stand apart from the "safe places" and tread in places of personal vulnerability. This kind of spiritual grounding precedes effective caregiving.

Preparedness for prayer, whether private or public, is therefore less about scripting than it is about shedding pretensions and harkening to the unknown and to the knowable. Where will the Divine take us? The Eternal One appears in our unguarded moments, prompting us to cry out silently or audibly for personal relief. In either case, our attentiveness is toward the pull of the Mystery. Every prayer is thus a "turning aside," an opening of self toward the Holy One as pain from underfoot shoots through the soul. The experience of Moses informs us that the most effective prayers are indeed God-ward as we feel the impact of thorns, sharp stones, bugs and bruises.

Grief, suffering, illness and death are the scorpions of our desert. If we do not feel the brokenness of our planet we have not yet had the holy experience. As we remove the sandals of clinical detachment from our caregiving we enter into the suffering of the Most High. The removal of sandals in sacred chronicles represents not only the healer's journey into God's pain, but also his/her shedding of status and self-protective defensiveness. When caregivers come to God and alongside patients with awareness of their own limitations and vulnerability, there is a shifting of feelings and perceptions. Prayers are no longer *for* patients but *with* patients. Prayer becomes more about *being* together than about *doing* for another.

In fact, the ultimate lesson of Moses' burning bush is this: any desiccated bush will glow with an inward strength and beauty when filled by the Sacred Other. This truth is both humbling and energizing. *Any* scraggly shrub will be transformed into an illuminating transformative force when it yields itself to the Divine Presence. As the spark of the Holy One enters, opportunities for both personal and systemic healing pop out at the right moment like blossoms of light in darkness.

FINDING SENSE IN FORTY CENTS

Lee, a hospital respiratory therapist, came grinning toward me and stopped me in the corridor. "I need to tell you a story. Do you have a minute?"

I nodded.

"Last month," he said, "our rent got jacked up unexpectedly and I've been worried. My income is frozen. Plus, my wife has been sick. So," he added, "I was complaining to God, thinking about Moses and how God provided for the Israelites when they were in the wilderness wandering between Egypt and Canaan."

Lee's complaints had been quite specific: "God, I hardly have two pennies to rub together. Are you listening, God? It would be nice to have even one penny for each of the 40 years that your servant Moses and the Israelites were in the desert. How about it, God? Do you hear me? I need help. Are you good for 40 cents?"

Lee said he had been despondent and anxious. So, he decided to take a mind-clearing walk down a long, sandy ocean shore. There he poured out his frustrations to a seemingly silent God.

Ocean waves had scrubbed the beach, erasing all footprints except those left behind by Lee. Face cast down, Lee's troubled eyes glanced ahead and fell upon a circular something resting upon the sand's surface. He reached down and plucked it from the sand. It was not a sand dollar, but a dime. Now ten cents richer, Lee continued his prayerful perambulations. "So, God, you're good for a dime..."

On and on down the trackless sand, Lee agonized in an open-eyed prayer for mercy. Then he found another coin – a quarter. Now 35 cents richer, Lee's spirits soared like gulls in a wave-whipped wind. "So, God, can you really take care of us? Can you give me five more cents as a sign?"

Lee's trek along the sandy expanse continued as he sought divine assurances. After placing another 100 feet of beach under his toes, Lee saw light bouncing up at him from another orb. It was a solitary nickel crying out to him. "In God we trust," it declared. The five cents joined the dime and quarter in Lee's hand, forming a witness to hope.

Sitting in the Waiting Place

The nurse's phone call came just as my shift was about to end. "Can you come and see Millie again? More family is here. They are asking for you." As I boarded the hospital elevator and ascended to Third Floor, I quickly replayed in my head an earlier conversation with Millie's husband. Their two sons had died at early ages from catastrophic illnesses. In their grief Rex and Millie had drawn closer together but more distant from their faith community. Still, prayer remained a precious coping resource for them. He had requested earlier that day that I come to sit and pray with him for a while. I did so until a crisis in the Emergency Department pulled me away. During that visit, he anticipated, as did the staff, that Millie would die within hours. Yet, six hours later, she was still "hanging on."

As I approached Millie's room, a middle-aged woman intercepted me and introduced herself as Julie, a niece of Rex and Millie. Pointing inside, she indicated that other cousins and friends had also come to say good-bye. "We've given her permission to go," she said. "So, we can't figure out what she's waiting for. It's been nearly two days now since she responded to anything or anyone. We've tried everything we can think of to reassure her. Would you come? Maybe another prayer will help?"

Just as I had earlier, I observed Rex sitting opposite the door near a window, ready to heed any signs of distress. I moved slowly around the foot of the bed and lowered myself beside him, positioning myself level with him so that I could easily see both his face and Millie's. "Tell me, Rex, a little more of your story. I know the two of you experienced some deep sorrow. Would you mind telling me more about how you rediscovered joy?"

Rex instantly smiled, and unpacked some delightful stories about a decade spent crisscrossing America in a motor home. "Those were good years. After we retired, we were able to spend all of our time together. We became vagabonds. We were truly footloose and fancy-free!"

"So," I pondered aloud, "I don't suppose you had a menagerie or zoo to feed?" He laughed and then grew quiet. "Actually, we have a dog," he said. "Out on the road we came across a puppy that adopted us. It was because of Charlie that we finally settled down. Charlie – that's his name – liked to ride in the back of the RV, looking out the rear window. But, it got to where every time a car or truck came up behind us he got agitated, scared and started barking. So, we listened to him. We quit the roads."

15

Suddenly, after a long pause, Rex said, "You know, I think Charlie is grieving."

At that moment, I glanced at Millie and saw her mouth twitching. Several times her facial muscles moved. Fascinated, I think, *something is stirring.* Looking at Rex, I continued our conversation, "Do you think God loves dogs?"

He responded, "Yes, I do. But, what do you think?"

"I think God *really* loves dogs," I said. "In fact, I think God has a *very* special place in his heart for dogs. And, I think God has at least two dogs."

Rex grinned quizzically. Time seemed to slow down as I looked at his Millie's face. Her eyelids and mouth were quivering with increased intensity. I continued to speak, asking Rex, "Do you know the Shepherd's Psalm?" (From my earlier visit, I knew he enjoyed reading his Bible though he and Millie had not attended church for many years).

Rex started quoting from memory, "The Lord is my Shepherd, I shall not want..." When he paused, I broke in, asking "What do you think? Do you suppose that a good sheep-herder might have a couple of good sheepdogs?" He grinned again.

Meanwhile, Millie's facial muscles were stretching. I kept my eyes fixed on her as Rex and I continued in unison, "Yea, though I walk through the valley of the shadow of death I will fear no evil for Thou art with me." On and on we recited! Toward the end I gestured for Rex to pause again. Looking at Millie, we could see that her eyes and mouth had stretched still more. I posed a question, "Rex and Millie, how does the Shepherd's Song end?"

Rex quoted from memory, "Surely, goodness and mercy shall follow me all the days..."

I gently interjected, "Stop right there! Again, what does it say? Do you see the Good Shepherd's dogs' names?"

Our eyes riveted on Millie, and her eyes opened wide, twinkling at us as we say together, "Goodness and Mercy!" A wide grin stretched across Millie's face as I paraphrased the story. "Can we say that in the valley of the shadow of death, the Good Shepherd sends his sheep dogs, Goodness and Mercy, to bring Millie into a good place?"

Millie's face was animated; her eyes glimmered and her mouth smiled though her body was very still and her breathing was labored. Rex and I completed the Shepherd's Song together. "And I will dwell in the House of the Lord forever." Slowly, slowly Millie's arms rose up from her bed sheets; her gnarled fingers stretched out to grip the hands of her husband of 56 years as I asked, "Millie, do you trust that God will take care of Charlie, and that his sheep dogs, Goodness and Mercy, will bring you into a good place?"

In response, Millie wordlessly directed a huge tender smile and sparkling eyes toward Rex as she peacefully in that moment released the final breath of her nomadic journey. The wait is over now. Goodness and Mercy, heaven's sheepdogs, came, and I was their witness.

STANDING IN A LAUGHING PLACE

One day as I walked down a long corridor between hospital units, I saw a woman approaching me. When she got closer our eyes met. Instantly she stumbled, caught herself, and suddenly stopped, groping for words as she greeted me: "You? You're alive! I can't believe it! You are…alive!"

As her jaw dropped, I puzzled over her words, trying to place her face. Where and when had we met? And WHY did she think I was dead? Tugging on my arm, she exclaimed, "Please! You must come! My sister thinks you're dead. Come!"

"Sure, I'm with you," I said, still wondering how this woman and her sister knew me. The lady promptly pivoted and escorted me a short distance to a doorway where she paused and motioned for me to enter ahead of her. A frizzy-haired woman sat beside her hospital bed. She glanced up, saw my face, and I then heard an echo: "You're alive! I can't believe it! You're alive!" Tears formed in her eyes and spilled down her cheeks as she smiled and laughed.

I too was grinning. I now remembered Sally, the patient, and Maria, her sister. I had met them when Sally came for heart surgery months earlier. At their request, I had prayed with them just before Sally's operation began, and then afterward while relaying progress reports to family members at critical junctures throughout the long day. We had then shared laughter, tears, and more prayers as Sally traveled the painful road to recovery. My conversations with her elderly parents were especially memorable. Their devout love for God and family touched a chord in my own heart, reminding me of my own parents.

"So you thought I was dead?" I said.

"Yes. We heard you died," they said in unison. Sally added, "We've got to call Mom and Dad! They were *very* sad when you died."

But, I wasn't dead!

"So, tell me why you thought I died," I said.

"Mom saw you on the news. The reporter said 'a much-loved person' at the hospital had a sudden heart attack and died. She saw your picture on TV."

Instantly I understood the source of her confusion. Yes, my face had appeared one night in a short news hiccup. In fact, a death had occurred at my hospital. But, the death was not mine. The occasion was the sudden death of a beloved physician. A reporter had interviewed me regarding how chaplains were providing support for grieving staff. That day, within the span of a 10 second sound bite, I went from being a breathing chaplain to being a dead man in the minds of Maria and her family.

"Mom and Dad have been going to church every morning to light candles and pray for your soul," Sally said. "I've got to phone them!"

"Wow! I'm grateful! Please give them my thanks, and tell them that their prayers have been heard! I am very much alive," I said.

My own perspective of happiness in those moments shifted. As Sally and Maria welcomed me back from the dead, I instantly sensed a parallel joy in heaven, the happy energy that the Holy One feels when His struggling creation responds to the reality of His Living Presence. As happy tears streamed down Sally and Maria's faces, suddenly my own joy erupted in waves of laughter. "Yes! I am alive! AND I am glad that YOU are glad that I am alive!" Backing out of the room with smiles and laughter, I wondered, "Will laughter be contagious today?"

18

TOASTING THE MIND

Sometimes I laugh so that I don't cry. Mom's mind has become a mysterious collage of wispy fuzz. Her husband Bob is now "that special guy." She doesn't remember his name but knows that he is her "Honey" and "Sweetheart." She knows that they've been together for "a long time," but can't tell you that it has been 65 years since she and Dad tied the knot on June 15, not long after Dad got back from "the war."

Now in her dotage, her questions are still the Who, What, When, Where, Why and How of the inquiring mind. But answers slip into the holes in the cheese that her mind has become. Five minutes after hearing an answer, she repeats herself. She will look for answers anywhere and everywhere.

An evening newsman smiles out at her from the flat screen TV. She's pleased. She loves smiles. But when she tries to start a conversation with news pundits like Charlie Gibson, her frustration surfaces. "What's wrong with him?" she asks me. "He needs to come out from behind that 'thing' and talk to us directly. He's just plain rude!" Through the years, Mom's propensity to fit people, places and things into compartments of her loving heart and brilliant mind has served her well. But now she struggles to make sense of how her world has changed.

Yet, there is a constant: She still wants to be useful. She still wants to help out however she can. Even now she exudes good will. She will gladly empty the dishwasher and cheerfully sort and organize the silverware – again and again and again and again all day long. She will fold the laundry meticulously hour after hour – refolding and refolding and refolding, aligning each seam precisely. And then she'll do it again. There's just one problem. She doesn't recognize whether she is emptying a dirty dishwasher or a clean one. She doesn't know if she's folding clean or soiled linen.

Then there is the matter of food, the longtime pride of Mom's fiefdom. After years of cooking and baking semi-gourmet meals for family, she embraced the KISS philosophy of meal preparation: Keep it Simple, Silly. Simply stated, Mom now loves toast.

Not long ago Mom awakened ahead of the household – my caregiving sister Sue and her husband Lee – and started breakfast preparations. Sue entered the kitchen and found Mom hovering over the toaster. A fragrance filled the air that seemed peculiar. Five times Mom had filled the toaster, and patiently awaited the emergence of the perfect slice. Yet, five times the toast was flawed. It just "didn't come out right."

As Mom bemoaned her failure to "get it right," Sue extracted the latest rendition: It was not bread but a perfectly folded pair of adult diapers. Five charred diapers in the garbage and one yet in the toaster testified to the frustrations of living on an aging planet.

Diapers. Kitchen barricades. Plastic-covered mattresses. Baby monitors on night stands. Do we laugh at Mom or with her? She does not know what she does. So, our laughter is filled with grief. Like a little child she is led to the breakfast nook where a meal is placed before her. She is fading and our pain is real. We grieve because we care. And we laugh because Mom has shared so much of her good heart with us, teaching us that there are values that transcend burned toast.

Having the Difficult Conversations

Many people feel uncomfortable just talking about dying. Even though death is inevitable they avoid speaking about it. And it is not easy to go against ancient and modern taboos. Yet, conversations about the "unthinkable" may bring relief to emotional distress and raw fear. In fact, talking about this topic may provide immeasurable benefits almost immediately and certainly for the long term. These conversations can bring a kind of wellness that overcomes the difficulties of the immediate crisis.

Ironically, even as global news media conveys the brutality of endless wars and the entertainment industry presents death in increasingly graphic ways, death remains a remote and difficult topic of conversation for many people. As society has shifted from agricultural communities to urban centers, values have become increasingly individualized, secularized, consumerized and technology-driven. Accordingly, caregivers are often called to help people move beyond "sound bite" summations of life and death to rediscover what truly matters. Having conversations about death, dying and grief strips away anonymity and restores the intimacy of deep personal caring.

Unfortunately, many people have lost the capacity and vocabulary to talk about death and related issues. The specialization and compartmentalization of care by experts has created its own vocabulary that is often different from what care recipients know and speak. It is therefore often our task as caregivers to help others find language that bridges over the incomprehensible into places of insight and spiritual awakening. This often happens as death threatens.

We provide care in a world that is polarized by various beliefs, and values, necessitating personal clarity of purpose and sensitivity toward diversity. Roy Disney, co-founder of Disney World, once said, "It is not hard to make decisions when we know our values." We approach end-of-life conversations with recognition that we are entering tunnels of the unknown where pirates of our emotions sing to us, "It's a small, small world…" We are called to humbly enter that small thin space where life and death intersect and to be attentive toward what really matters in those days, hours, or moments. Only in self-awareness and Spirit-cognition will our conversations have outcomes that are satisfactory to both caregiver and care recipient. Identification of values is the starting point for end-of-life conversations. These values often emerge when persons are facing their mortality.

GIVING BAD NEWS – SEVEN EMPATHIC PAUSES

Physicians are usually the first persons to deliver bad news. And often it is a repetitive process that involves a whole team. Whoever the bad-news-bearer is, it is not an easy task. Never should the process be treated lightly, and ideally, it should not be rushed.

When emergencies compel a doctor to dash elsewhere, continued support is vital. Empathic physicians will hand off support to other team members to attend to the emotional chaos that has just been triggered. Often the bad news must be phrased and then rephrased, again and again. Chaplains and other trained persons can assist doctors with this process.

When presenting difficult news to patients and family members, it is important to think ahead not only about what will be said, but how to say it. Here are some basic guidelines for when it is necessary to speak "hard truths":

1. Pause to strategize with the care team. Before approaching the patient and family, take time to ensure that someone will be alongside to support during *and* after bad news is delivered.

2. Pause with the patient and family to identify what is understood and what isn't. For example, "What is your understanding of what is happening?" Listen carefully for indicators of poor comprehension and/or underlying fears that may be impeding an ability to fully hear what is actually happening.

3. Pause, then kindly warn the patient and/or family that they will now hear something that may be very upsetting. For example, "I am sorry that I must tell you something that may be painful to hear."

4. Pause again so that the patient and/or family can compose their emotions and prepare themselves for what they are now about to hear. And then, deliver the news with short, simple sentences. For example, "Your mother's heart is very tired and weak; it is struggling to pump blood; the poor blood-flow is now affecting other parts of her body. Her kidneys and lungs are shutting down..."

5. Pause to allow time for each person to take in and start processing the bad news.

6. Pause to allow time for persons to verbalize their questions and fears. Then, answer them compassionately and honestly. If there are no clear answers, say so clearly.

7. Pause to acknowledge emotions and to assure non-abandonment: "This is a hard time. No matter what lies ahead, I want you to know that I am here to walk alongside you, to support you in whatever way feels right for you. If I am not here, one of my colleagues will be available..." Utilizing and affirming a team approach is more helpful than making promises that we might not be able to keep.

In these encounters two values are essential: honesty and kindness. When we are with persons traumatized by bad news or hard choices, we join with them in a journey. The reality may be so horrific that it exceeds our imaginations. Yet, we speak it honestly: "Your son was killed this morning," "You have Stage 4 terminal cancer," "We've exhausted all treatment options," "You are dying." When death is imminent or has just happened, it is no time for sugar-coating truth. Saccharine euphemisms can contribute to avoidance rather than acceptance of reality, and may mask kindness rather than reveal it.

Honesty without kindness is cruelty. Thus, *before* we speak, God calls us to listen inwardly, seeking the Abiding Source of healing and hope. We let the Sacred One's empathy rise from our hearts to our eyes, ears, and lips and face. Listening, seeing, speaking and emoting, we convey hope. We move forward in incremental baby steps alongside care recipients, allowing the ultimate outcome to reveal itself without anyone or anything being rushed.

In these interactions, it is important to remember that not all values are religiously informed or structured. Thus, when talking about end-of-life concerns, even while we strategize, it is important to know that the pre-scripting (prior scripting) of a conversation or an outcome can get in the way of identifying the nature and origin of personal values, thereby thwarting access to a person's inner self.

Emotional and spiritual pain is often related to how one's values have been shaped and challenged. Such pain is deeply personal. Thus, when talking with most people, it is important, I believe, to approach them with the language of daily living rather than the language of piety, spirituality and religion. One way to do this is by looking at quality-of-life issues.

As spiritual caregivers, we acknowledge that sometimes we reach the point where medical interventions are no longer prolonging life. Instead they are extending an unnatural and unacceptable quality of life by refusing to heed what body, mind and spirit are indicating.

In person-centered caregiving, it is ethically imperative that individual values not be negated by technological possibilities (or caregivers' well-intended agendas). For this reason, I collaborated with an interdisciplinary team of co-workers to create a simple questionnaire to facilitate quality-of-life conversations between caregivers and family members. It is used primarily when a loved one has become incapable of voicing his/her own desires. However, the tool's open-ended questions and statements may be modified for usage also with lucid, communicative patients, or for self-evaluation among caregivers. While it may be placed in the hands of hospital patrons to complete at their leisure or not, it may also simply serve as an internal lens to ascertain the nature of a person's core spirituality. I recommend Dr. Richard Groves' book, "The American Book of Dying" for additional insights into spiritual assessments at end of life.

What I want to know as I approach an end-of-life situation can be summarized in variations of one question: "How are you within?" Once trust is established, it is a question I may pose to a dying person or to that person's family members. By posing the question, I acknowledge the reality of mortality and invite the entrance of hope.

When we are not able to deliver a cure for death, I know that a kind of healing is happening when I ask, "How are you within?" and the dying or grieving person is able to say, "I am well." The miracle of this kind of wellness is larger than death. Being witness to this is our privilege as caregivers.

Wellness is connected to both quality of life and hope. So, here are some tools to help facilitate conversations. The first is the Quality-of-Life Self-Assessment Tool that I just mentioned. The second is the script of a brochure about Cardio-Pulmonary Resuscitation (CPR). Without using religious jargon, both help persons focus on what is truly important when facing end-of-life decisions.

When utilizing the quality-of-life tool, one can total up the eight numeric scores to establish a baseline for monitoring how well we are attending to a person's core values and needs. A higher score indicates greater resiliency and coping resources. A lower score indicates a need to talk further about how plans of care can be aligned with the patient's wishes. (See page 179 for a scoring rubric.)

Take a few minutes to practice with the tool. Apply it first to yourself and then go through it with someone else whom you know well, perhaps with a family member. This process allows us to tune our hearts more closely to the heart of others. By placing ourselves in the patient's circumstances, we become more patient-centered in our caregiving. The outcome we then seek become more life-honoring whether the end is life or death.

A *QUALITY-OF-LIFE ASSESSMENT TOOL*

Quality-of-Life Assessment
For a Cognitively Impaired Family Member

Instructions: Help us to know your loved one. In each of the areas below circle the number or word that most closely describes your loved one. Try to answer from the patient's point of view.

Healthy Purpose

1. The patient finds meaning and purpose in his/her life:

1	2	3	4	5	6
Rarely	*Seldom*	*Occasionally*	*Sometimes*	*Usually*	*Always*

2. What brings joy and purpose to him/her?
    How important is that to him/her?

1	2	3	4	5	6
Not at all important				*Extremely important*	

Healthy Relationships

3. The patient feels closely connected to family and friends:

1	2	3	4	5	6
Rarely	*Seldom*	*Occasionally*	*Sometimes*	*Usually*	*Always*

4. Who (or what) does the patient need in order to feel at peace?
    How important is that to the patient?

1	2	3	4	5	6
Not at all important				*Extremely important*	

Healthy Expectations

5. The patient is hopeful about his/her future:

1	2	3	4	5	6
Rarely	*Seldom*	*Occasionally*	*Sometimes*	*Usually*	*Always*

6. Who/what contributes to your loved one's emotional and spiritual well-being? How important are those resources to the patient?

1	2	3	4	5	6
Not at all important				*Extremely important*	

Healthy Body

7. The patient is able to accept and enjoy life even with physical and/or mental limitations.

1	2	3	4	5	6
Rarely	*Seldom*	*Occasionally*	*Sometimes*	*Usually*	*Always*

8. What is essential to sustain your loved one's desire to live? _____
    How important is that to your loved one?

1	2	3	4	5	6
Not at all important				*Extremely important*	

Tips For Decision-Making
When the Heart is Struggling

Cardiopulmonary Resuscitation (CPR) is the process of attempting to restart the heart. It is a serious procedure which may not be beneficial for everyone.

Here is a question to ask yourself: Do you want to be resuscitated when near the end of life? This question concerns what to do if the heart stops or if one cannot breathe. In other words, if your heart stops, do you want to be revived?

When a person is in an advanced diseased state or approaching the end of life, it is important to be aware of the following facts:

- **Not choosing is actually a choice.** *By default, according to the law in most areas, healthcare professionals must attempt to revive you or your loved one by whatever means necessary if wishes are not clearly known. It is the care team's responsibility to tell you what your options are and their implications, and it is your responsibility to make your wishes clear. Though this is a painful subject for many, it can be more painful if it is ignored.*

  A sobering fact: While CPR can extend the length of life, it can also extend the dying process while increasing suffering. Quality of life may be significantly diminished.

  Many people find it useful to speak to their doctor about what to expect if they choose to be revived with CPR. Your doctor can explain what happens and how life may be different afterwards.

- **CPR is not a simple choice.** *CPR has become increasingly complex as healthcare professionals have expanded their knowledge, methods, and efforts to prolong life. Unless told to do otherwise, emergency responders may use strong drugs and other interventions along with chest compressions. Choosing CPR during a cardiac arrest may also*

26

result in being placed on a ventilator (breathing machine) for the rest of one's life.

- **CPR can extend life, but life can be radically different afterwards**. *CPR does not always work as it appears on television and in the movies. Entertainment media brings patients back to life 75% of the time. It leads people to think that a majority of CPR recipients return home (Diem, et al 1998).*

  But in real life, at best only about 17% of otherwise healthy persons go home from the hospital (Peberdy, et al 2003). Patients who are seriously ill in Acute Care and Intensive Care have an even lower probability of returning home. Those who do survive may require lengthy recovery periods in rehabilitation facilities or nursing homes.

  A sobering fact: When CPR brings a person back to life, the chance of that person going home with the same brain function is about 7% (Kaldjian, et al 2009).

- **CPR is an uncomfortable experience**. *During a Code Blue (cardiac arrest and/or cessation of breathing), the interdisciplinary team strives to treat the patient with respect and dignity. However, personal space and privacy is invaded. Chest compressions can result in damage to the rib cage, lungs and windpipe. As multiple specialists converge at the patient's bedside, family members are usually unable to be alongside their loved one while he/she is perhaps dying. This can intensify grief.*

- **CPR often results in broken bones**. *Persons with degenerative bone disease, oncology patients whose bone structure has been compromised by radiation, and the elderly are especially vulnerable. For those who survive a heart stoppage, extended CPR can also diminish brain functioning.*

- **Personal values shape our living and our dying**. *The CPR decision is ultimately about much more than receiving or accepting a treatment option. It really is about how we choose to live. Some may choose to accept all life-saving measures. Others will choose to not have CPR performed. Whatever the decision and whatever the reasons, the care* team is committed to treating each person with respect and dignity. It is therefore important to make your wishes known.

- **Life's best decisions include end-of-life planning.**
  The CPR decision is just part of a larger picture that includes all that brings meaning and purpose to each day. As death approaches, it is not uncommon for people to say that their lives have been enriched even as their bodies are shrinking. Life becomes increasingly precious and focused as it starts to fade. During this time, it is important to ask these questions:
  - When death comes, whom do you want to be with?
  - Where is your ideal place to die?
  - What would bring resolution to unresolved emotional and spiritual pain?
  - With your decisions, are you prolonging life or extending the dying process?
  - What do you need to say and/or hear in order to know that your life is ending well.

By making your wishes known in advance, you increase the likelihood that you will be able to live and die the way you want, surrounded by those you love.

For support in your decision-making, please call a chaplain. We are committed to providing emotional and spiritual care in ways that are respectful of personal values, needs and wishes.

The Finish Line

When we care deeply, we feel enormous tension between hanging on and letting go, especially at the end of life. We therefore want to acknowledge the heartache that comes when we prepare to say good-bye.

Clinically trained chaplains are available to walk alongside you, helping you to find hope and the power to cope as you navigate through difficult times. You may contact a chaplain by calling the hospital operator or asking any staff member for a chaplain's visit.

Chaplain Services

Our Mission: to help patients, families, and staff find hope and the power to cope by caring for spiritual and religious needs in ways that honor personal wishes and choices.

References:

Diem, S. J., J. D. Lantos, and J. A. Tulsky. 1996. Cardiopulmonary Resuscitation on Television: Miracles and Misinformation. New England Journal of Medicine 334 (24): 1578–82.

Kaldjian, L.C., Z.D. Erekson, T.H. Haberle, et al. 2009. Code Status Discussion and Goals of Care Among Hospitalized Adults. Journal of Medical Ethics 35 (6): 338–42.

Peberdy, M.A., W. Kaye, J.P. Ornato, et al. 2003. Cardiopulmonary Resuscitation of Adults in the Hospital: A report of 14,720 cardiac arrests from the National Registry of Cardiopulmonary Resuscitation. Resuscitation 58 (3): 297–308.

The research referenced in the above brochure script was found on the website of Viki Kind, a bioethicist who specializes in end-of-life-decision issues. For further information on this and other topics, I recommend this link (http://kindethics.com/2010/09/10-pitfalls-to-avoid-in-dnr-decision-making) and her website (http://www.thecaregiverspath.com).

TRIAGING PAIN AND GRIEF

Managing emotions while in the midst of end-of-life situations can be challenging. Toss love in the air like a coin, and the face that appears in the palm of your hand may be pain or anger. Some days are slower than others. But, sometimes the painful "stuff" pours down faster and with more force than we can catch or hold. As caregivers, our capacity to function effectively is tied to our ability to juggle multiple assaults on our senses. These pressures may be such that we nearly suffocate from emotional and physical exhaustion. How can we survive relentless waves of pain? No time to run to the chapel! No time to voice more than a "God, have mercy!" Barely time to breathe!

Sometimes a tsunami of grief hits with not just one wave, but a seemingly endless series of rogue bone-breakers. As you continue to read, please look and listen to the tremors beneath and between the waves. Where does this one day, this one eight-hour shift, take you within yourself? How do you triage in such circumstances? How do you navigate in and around currents of grief without suffocating? (Be aware: not every day is like this, but some are.)

6:30 a.m.   The morning shift is just starting. I have just entered the office and am taking off my coat. The desk phone rings. It is from the nighttime hospital supervisor regarding an unfolding situation in Room 1040. A 34 year-old mother of four small children has had a massive stroke apparently caused by a sudden dissecting carotid artery. Brain death is likely. Considerations: how to emotionally and spiritually support this large non-English speaking family; how to facilitate the organ donor requestor process; how staff, some of whom are young mothers, might experience this death; how to prioritize. I clip my cell phone and pager to my belt and head out.

6:40 a.m.   A patient is about to undergo open-heart surgery. Twice I will meet with the patient's family to provide progress reports from the cardio-vascular operating room. I give the patient and his family a brief pre-op orientation regarding how, when, and where I will deliver information to the family.

6:50 a.m.   The Organ Procurement Agency (OPA) phones, seeking my assessment of how the organ requesting process should proceed for the woman in 1040.

7:00 a.m.   I consult with ICU staff about the patient in 1040 and then call the OPA back, telling them that we will be having a Family Care Conference later after a second brain scan confirms the brain death. I hang up and immediately feel the phone vibrating again, alerting me to a message that has entered my voice mailbox while I've been talking. I access it.

7:15 a.m.   An ICU nurse tells me that the wife of a patient in 1030 is distraught and wants a chaplain to come see her as soon as possible. As I approach the room, I pass by 1028 where a patient and his wife gesture for me to come in. Our visit is brief, with expressions of mutual gratitude for the success of yesterday's open-heart surgery. I move on and am visiting with the patient who's requested my visit when my cell phone vibrates.

7:25 a.m.   The ICU manager tells me that a patient in 1006 is in crisis. Again, it is a young mother in her 30s. Her brain has experienced a traumatic injury following surgery to remove a foreign object left accidentally in her body three years earlier during surgery in a developing country. Like the young mother in 1040, this intubated mother of four will also die soon, perhaps today, if a miracle does not occur. I check in with her nurse. The family has left to get breakfast while staff does bedside assessments and testing. I inform the nurse that I will return later when family is present.

Just one hour has passed since my shift began. Already two rooms, two dying mothers, each about to leave behind four children – a total of eight! The cell phone vibrates again.

7:45 a.m.   A man has just died in 1034 after seven weeks in intensive care following a single-car accident while returning from his nighttime work as a janitor at a bank. (His adult children from a previous marriage have told me that the patient's young wife was having an affair.) His wife is now en route to the hospital, coming from a neighboring town. I wonder, how will the dead man's older adult children and his second family of three pre-adolescent children manage their grief? Have they all been contacted? Also, how will staff cope with the death of someone who has been so long under their care? Will I need to arrange a debriefing session for staff?

Three rooms, three different parents, a total of eleven young children whose world is being turned upside down!

7:50 a.m.   My cell phone vibrates. The intensivist will be meeting with the family of 1040 for a family care conference at about 8:15, would I please join them? I look at my watch: 25 minutes until the meeting starts. I have time for at least one more visit, maybe more if the care conference is late, as often happens.

7:55 a.m.   I go to the deceased man's room, 1034, where I stand quietly at the bedside, silently praying and remembering moments of seeing his eloquent tears while assisting his non-verbal communication with his adult children during frequent long-distance phone "conversations." He has demonstrated several times to me that those in a coma are yet "at home." Now he is beyond his coma. Around his neck is an amethyst crucifix placed there by his heavily tattooed adult son. He wants it left on him for his cremation, but wonders if the young stepmother will allow it. That wife is still on her way to the hospital from out of town. I wonder, can I set my judgments aside?

8:00 a.m.   I head toward 1040. I am concerned about how the patient's nurse, a new mother herself, will deal with the challenges of caring for the dying 30 year-old mother of four. When I check in with her, she says she's okay, but is aware of emotions being stirred. We then talk about the patient and her family before I enter the patient's room. Though the family's English is limited, I am able to establish a connection with the father and his brother before our soon-to-start Family Care Conference with Dr. Jones. I confirm that the family's request for a priest was met during the night. I seek and receive permission to join them when they meet with the doctor. I let them know that our 8:15 meeting will likely start a little late.

8:15 a.m.   I go to the ICU lobby to confirm that the open-heart patient's family is present for upcoming reports. At the same time, I meet with additional family members of the patient in 1040, and put some of them in one of the hospital's Family Conference Rooms.

8:30 a.m.   I am now two hours into my shift. I unlock the ICU Conference Room and escort 1040's family there from the lobby and the patient's bedside. I briefly facilitate introductions of the interdisciplinary team and our meeting begins. Dr. Jones guides the family through the medical scenario, outlining the likely outcome. It is an emotionally intense 45 minutes as the family struggles to process and absorb what they hear through a professional interpreter. I am aware of religious and cultural nuances that are shaping their questions and responses. Where appropriate I seek clarification of wishes and needs. A decision is made to reconvene later in the day to reevaluate the direction of care. After the doctor and other staff leave, I remain with the family a while longer, validating their emotions and affirming our availability for ongoing support. They are a deeply spiritual family and begin talking about how we are each a part of the body of Christ. The Lord, they say, is in charge. I am aware that as part of that body, I am feeling their pain. I leave to talk with the lead nurse regarding contact with the Organ Procurement Agency.

9:15 a.m.   My cell phone vibrates. It is an outside call from a member of our chaplaincy team. I am asked to check in with staff in the Neonatal Intensive Care Unit where there is a brain dead infant. The issue: Is the family actually needing and requesting a Protestant Spanish-speaking chaplain or do they want a Catholic priest to support them? Triaging, I ask my colleague to call directly to the NICU's pediatric social worker for clarification. As I hang up, my cell phone vibrates again. It is the ICU unit secretary calling me from 15 feet away wanting to connect me with a floor nurse who simultaneously sees me from her location just down the corridor. She hastens toward me, an expression of relief on her face. "Please! I need you. The wife [of 1034] is here! She's hysterical and she's got three small crying children with her!" I accompany the nurse into the room, encountering waves of loud moaning and wailing. The distraught wife collapses in my arms. The children look on with tearful, fearful faces. I am now nearly three hours into my shift.

9:25 a.m.   I am paged from the operating room with a report for waiting family members. The heart patient is now on the heart-lung machine, otherwise known as "the pump." But, I choose to stay with the newly widowed wife and fatherless children in 1034, postponing my report to the open-heart patient's family until this death scene's traumatized emotions are eased. I engage the deceased patient's wife in conversation, eliciting stories, gradually shifting her attention toward her children. She sobs, "I don't know how I can replace him!" In a few minutes a social worker enters. I hand off the mom's care to her. I kneel on the floor and engage the children in their grief responses. Their emotions are raw as we talk about how they've fished and hiked with their dad. We talk about ways in which they will remember their father.

10:15 a.m.   My phone vibrates periodically – a call from Organ Procurement, a call from a nurse who is with a family member who is "sobbing uncontrollably," a call from the print shop. At last, I excuse myself from 1034 for a short while to triage and to relay the surgical report to the heart patient's family. Reentering 1034, the three small children once again surround me. A seven-year old boy's red-haired head is pressed against my leg, his arms embracing me. Tears pool in his eyes as I kneel down in front of him, holding him, his moist cheek against mine. The oldest child, a 10-year-old boy, offers me his New Testament as the family gathers at the bedside. We read several Bible promises from the child's Bible, have prayer together, and then I assist the wife with some final paperwork. When all is done, her small children remain clinging to my legs. They gaze into my face with tear-filled eyes as their mother walks toward the elevator, calling back to them, telling them that it's time to go. I hug them quickly – three small fatherless children. As they disappear through the corridor toward the elevator, the overhead intercom announces a trauma code in the emergency department. My shift is not yet half over.

11:15 a.m.   A freight train has clipped an elderly couple's car at 50 mph. While the wife is being coded in ED #36, the husband is being treated in ED #24. I shuttle between the two rooms, tag-teaming with Ivan, a social worker, to find family contact information, and assess other needs.

11:45 a.m.   My phone vibrates. A nurse says that a hospital volunteer's oldest son is undergoing emergent cardiac catheterization. "The wife is pretty emotional. Can you come right away?" I explain that I am still involved in an ED code and will come as soon as I can.

11:50 a.m.   Five minutes later, my pager buzzes and I hear an overhead announcement of another Code Blue, this time in Room 256 on Surgical Floor. After consultation with the hospital supervisor, I transfer care of the ED patients, the husband and wife, to the ED's social worker and dash across the hospital.

12 noon   Just as I arrive at the new code site, I am paged by the Cardio-vascular Operating Room and am told that the heart patient is now "off-pump." Her heart is now beating on its own. I defer delivering the report and remain with the Code Blue situation until the elderly man is stabilized.

12:30 p.m.   The hospital supervisor, clears me to leave the code. I return to the ICU lobby and deliver a report to the heart patient's family.

12:40 p.m.   I backtrack to the other side of the hospital to locate the family of the emergent cardiac catheterization patient. The anxious family is now supported by their pastor, all of them seeking information. In the heart catheterization lab, I find that the procedure is finished, the patient is doing well, and the cardiac interventionist will soon talk with family. I relay this information, leaving the family in the care of their pastor.

1:00 p.m.   I boot up my computer and start documenting morning visits, codes and care conferences while eating lunch at my desk.

1:15 p.m.   I receive a phone call from the birth center. A patient has had a fetal demise. "Not an immediate need, but the family would like a visit when you can get here. They'll be here for a while. So, don't rush." I don't.

1:30 p.m.   The evening shift chaplain arrives. I hand off the fetal demise request, as well as support for a second open heart patient and follow-up of the family in 1006. Just as I am about to hand over the pager and cell phone to my colleague, the phone vibrates once more. It is a nurse in the Clinical Decision Unit (CDU) relaying a patient's request "for Chaplain Tom." Now free of the cell phone and pager, I head to CDU. As I enter the patient's room I recognize her from a previous lengthy hospitalization. Mental health issues intersect with abuse issues. I hear a litany of woes – some familiar to me, many sounding quite rehearsed.

2:30 p.m.   My usual departure time! End of shift! I am back in the office, finished with my charting. My coat is on and I'm ready to leave. The desk phone rings. Do I answer it or not? It is the Organ Procurement Team. They ask for an update regarding how and when to approach the family of the brain-dead mother of four in 1040. I give them what I know and then hang up. Immediately the desk phone rings again. I am informed by a nurse that 1040's doctor is calling an immediate care conference to share new brain scan results. The doctor is quite clear: He does not want to deliver bad news without a chaplain. Knowing that my chaplain colleague is dealing with the fetal demise, I cannot hand off to her. So, I respond though my shift is over. During the Care Conference, family members are seemingly too numb to fully absorb the reality that the young mother is now actually legally dead though her heart yet beats. There are no brain waves. Her pupils no longer respond to any stimuli. When the doctor briefly breaks protocols and introduces the idea of organ donation, I sense that it is too early to further pursue this topic. Emotions are too raw. Following the Family Care Conference I consult further with interdisciplinary team members about our next steps. I will remain available to return to the hospital to support the family when they are asked further about organ donation. I leave my personal contact information at the nursing station.

3:45 p.m.   Back in our office, I reboot my computer and document the care conference. I then phone Organ Procurement, updating them once again, and giving them my personal contact information in case I need to return to the hospital to be with the family when they are approached about donating their loved one's organs.

4:00 p.m.   While exiting the hospital, I poke my head into the office of my hospital supervisor and update her regarding the organ donation process for the young mother who is brain dead in 1040. In this context, we also talk about the plethora of physician and staff-referred patients and families who are yet unvisited throughout the hospital. I share with her that I did not make it to Medical, Surgical, Pediatrics, NICU, the Birth Center, Inpatient Rehab, or Oncology. I have handed all of that off to my evening colleague.

4:15 p.m.   There is still daylight. I depart for home.

If one day is so brutal, how can I return day after day, year after year without burning out? Repetitive experiences with despair and human brokenness inform me that I need repetitive doses of hope. I need reliable, quickly accessible resources to replenish my inner-self when daily pressures are sucking the air out of me. What sustains me when waves of pain and grief come so quickly at me that I feel that I am drowning?

Eons ago I was trained to be a lifeguard. I remember my instructor saying that if I was ever caught in an ocean current pulling me away from shore, I should not fight it, but should instead spread my body across the water's surface and let myself be carried for a while. While I conserved energy, he said, the ocean might transport me along the shore to a place where it might deposit me on safe ground again with far less of my strength being consumed. Work with the currents, he said, rather than against them.

Likewise in caregiving, ongoing vitality depends on how well we are able to let go of a compass that is not working, and yield to one that does. How does one let go of suffocating grief and pain?

From my childhood, I believe I was being equipped to do the work that I do today, being gradually taught some secrets of self-care. In our home we had a Friday night ritual. We gathered as a family to individually share the ups-and-downs of our week. Sometimes we played games together; sometimes we read stories together. Then, we children all went to bed between freshly washed, sun-dried sheets to bask in an awareness of our parent's love. Clean sheets filled my nostrils with the scent of peace and rest. To this day as I climb between clean linen, I am often transported into a sacred story taught me by Mom and Dad. It is a story that I turn to internally as I dash from crisis to crisis. The story wraps itself around me and carries me when I am disintegrating emotionally, physically and spiritually. It tells me who I am and how much I am loved.

Managing Chaos

Join me in the ancient Book of Origins, otherwise known as the Book of Genesis. It opens with a description of an earth that was "formless and void." There was just emptiness and darkness (Genesis 1:1, 2, *NIV*). This early picture is not unlike the emotional landscape of my life when I am beaten down, pulverized and depleted. I feel compelled to know what God does with this chaos.

First, God shows up. Then, like a musician setting a metronome in motion, he sets a tempo for His creation. His first note is, "Let there be light," signaling that into darkness comes hope. Immediately His Holy Breath moves in and around the chaos, working to transform emptiness into fullness, and chaos into tranquility. God's baton goes up and down, circling seven times.

In six days, God created heaven and earth, pausing repeatedly to say, "It is good!" The final pause is longer. On the eve of the sixth day, God signals the start of a full, complete stop, a full day during which a single tone pulsates throughout the new creation; it is the heartbeat of heaven. Creation's Song starts with chaos and ends with a multi-dimensional crescendo of the Divine Presence. Dissonance yields to harmony. Wholeness births peace.

My heart yearns for this. Therefore, as I move throughout the hospital from crisis to crisis, I periodically, intentionally slow my footsteps and my breathing, pausing to listen internally and around me for the Orchestrator of Life. I apply brakes to the pace of body, mind and spirit in order to remember.

Pause with me and listen to the musical score of creation week; there is no proclamation of goodness on the first day. Observe the flow of music. When the Divine Troubadour enters, chaos shifts. Emptiness is no more. But, on the second, third, fourth and fifth days, God sings, "It's good." Then on the sixth day, there is once again a shift. the Mighty Maestro proclaims, "It is *very* good!" What is so good in this stanza of time that God says his creation is *very* good?

On the sixth day, "God created man in his own image, in the image of God he created him; male and female he created them" (Genesis 2:27, *NIV*). He did this because, "It is not good for man to be alone." The empty space, the void in Adam's life, was filled by a union of intimacy with the crowning creature of God's creation – woman. How good can this be? Humankind is special! Man and woman are precious, first shaped by God's own hands, and then breathed into by God's own mouth! They were designed intimately for intimacy!

As evening approaches and the seventh day begins, these two newly formed beings turn toward each other with recognition of a mystery. Eyes meet eyes. Face looks to face. Eyes survey the scenery. Hearts flip-flop in unison, engaging in the foreplay of discovery. Gravity pulls like toward like, love toward love. Otherness becomes oneness in an ecstatic outpouring of soul to soul, then comes the afterglow. Does she have a headache? Does he need Viagra? Do they sleep from exhaustion in love's aftermath? Indeed, who needs rest when one has the stamina of heaven's Eternal Breath? When life is so VERY good, who needs a break?

Yet, God rested! Consider, "By the seventh day God finished the work He had been doing; so on the seventh day he *rested* from all his work. And God blessed the seventh day and made it holy, because on it He *rested* from all the work of creating that he had done" (Genesis 2:1, 2, *NCV,* emphasis supplied).

There is a conundrum here. Why does God rest? Does God become tired? Certainly not! According to Judeo-Christian beliefs, God dwells in eternity. Therefore, he is beyond the vagaries of time, including exhaustion. He declares, "I the Lord do not change" (Malachi 3:6, *NIV*). Thus, I know that God's rest is not about depleted energy, but rather is somehow linked to the constancy of God's character.

Before the new creation was fractured by humankind's misuse of God-given free will, love and rest were different from what poses for love and rest today. That is true for both God and humankind. By forgetting God's intentions for humans and the Sabbath, grief is compounded. Thus, the call to remember! God summons us back to Eden both in Sabbath and in our relationships.

Tranquility and peace are expressions of God's transcendent nature and reliability. This is what God's rest day is all about! By resting *with* humankind the Creator provided a means whereby His innate, infinite peace and reliability move out of eternity into time and our finiteness. It is a repetitive stroke of genius. After breathing life into man and woman and overseeing their union on the sixth day, God breathed life into his newly formed world.

As our planet spins on its axis in relationship to light, we find that God's Sabbath is accessible and is filled with the Sacred Promise wherever we are! Even as the sun disappears into darkness, it promises that the True Light of Heaven who appeared in the realm of chaos and emptiness on the first day of creation is yet ours to fill all emptiness. The God of Righteousness will always reappear with healing in His voice and hands.

This renewal process is a mystery hinted at by some ancient words. Significantly, *Shabbos,* the Hebrew word for Sabbath, is tied to the word *yashab* that means, "to dwell." What this means is that the God who Sabbaths, or rests, with his creation is a God who *abides* with His creation. In other words, God descends into human time, injecting himself into the Sabbath. With God alongside, His sacred attributes push back against chaos, resulting in peace and harmony. In sharing His infinite self in a crescendo of companionship, God established a rejuvenating resource for all generations.

As I pause to remember and respond to God's presence, I feel my fragmented, disjointed self move toward reintegration through union with an energizing Presence. A sense of wholeness and renewal is gradually transmitted to me as my finite humanness yields to His infinite divinity.

Even as God partook of time, he invited his new creation to partake of his divine nature. There are non-transferable attributes of God that are uniquely God's own such as perfect foreknowledge. Yet there are other qualities or virtues that are transferred to us as we welcome His presence. Love, peace, joy, serenity, and eternal life – all these and more become a part of our being when we choose to be with God and remember the depths of His caring. Within Sabbath time/eternity we inhale the atmosphere of the Divine.

In a fractured world, what does this rest mean for the cancer patient whose cells are exploding out of control, multiplying and overpowering healthy cells, threatening to separate a young mother from her children? What does this mean to the widowed father whose son has just killed himself in a bout of depression after losing his job? What does this mean to the surgeon whose knowledge and best efforts are not enough to spare his own mother's life? When life spins out of control, how does God's Sabbath matter?

Here's how: It provides a landing place for us that cannot be taken away. It becomes a staircase that descends into and arises out of the crevasse of this world's brokenness. It links us to a past time when all was very good, and redirects and carries us toward a healing oasis on the horizon. It provides a bridge over troubled waters. It is a bridge with footings placed at creation on the Solid Rock of God's personhood.

Through the Sabbath, the Lord of the Sabbath makes this pledge: "'As the new heavens and the new earth that I make will endure before me,' declares the Lord, 'so will your name and your descendants endure. From one New Moon to another and from one Sabbath to another, all mankind will come and bow down before me,' says the Lord" (Isaiah 66:22, *NIV*). The Sabbath indeed means hope. The Sabbath means restoration of broken health and broken families. This is because it is a perpetual link to the God who cares.

Pain of the soul goes deep, taking many forms. There is pain from loss of meaning and purpose; there is pain from loss of connectedness to people, places, and activities; there is pain when forgiveness is needed; there is the pain of despair that may lead to suicide. Through His Sabbath, the Lord speaks to these issues, restoring identity, rebuilding relationships, bringing grace and hope. The Sabbath is God's weekly (and constant) reminder that God is present to re-integrate and renew our lives, both within us and around us. It shifts our spirits from "Oh no!" to "OHHHH! WOW!" It helps us catch our breath after being socked in the gut!

For several decades I lived among people who use a pictographic/ideographic script that dates back to the time of Abraham, Isaac, and Jacob. The Japanese word for Sabbath captures very well the essence of how God enters into this day and into our lives. Three ideographs are linked together in sequence to portray what Sabbath is all about. First is the character *an* (pronounced *ahn)* for "peace, serenity, and tranquility"; then comes the character *soku* which portrays "breath and spirit"; the third is *nichi,* the character for "day." *Ansokunichi* is thus the day in which Breath and Spirit bring peace, serenity, and tranquility. Concurrently, it is also the day in which peace eases breathing. The first character, *an,* can be also translated "ease." Thus, the day that breathes "ease" into us is the day that heals from dis-*ease.* Observance of creation week's Sabbath is very much about experiencing wholeness, healing, and life through relationship with the Creator.

REDIRECTING ENERGY

Obtaining the benefits of God's Sabbath is a discipline that involves a reordering of our energy and priorities. Our culture is driven by results, and our worth is often measured by how much we accomplish. Though this causes enormous performance anxieties, we remain outcome-oriented, striving to match or exceed ever-growing expectations. This is especially true in healthcare. We want to fix what is broken. We want to control our environment to guarantee our objectives. But, what happens when our efforts are not enough?

The answer to our pressure-cooker environment may be found not in working harder, but in working more wisely with a redirection of our energies. In the late first century a New Testament writer declared, "A Sabbath rest remains, therefore, for God's people. For the person who has entered His rest has rested from His own works, just as God did from His. *Let us then make every effort to enter that rest"* (Hebrews 4:9-11, *HCSB,* emphasis supplied).

The Lord of the Sabbath invites us to discipline ourselves to let go of our exhausting work-oriented, production mentality in favor of a God-directed way of being. He invites us to give up our "gotta-fix-this" mindset by yielding control to a trustworthy companion who is both Most High God and Most Nigh God. Transcendence and immanence, loftiness and nearness are hallmarks of God's nature. As we train our body, mind and spirit to "remember the Sabbath," we let go, granting God "breathing room" in us so that He can sort out our inner fragmentation and bring harmony to our being and doing. One Sabbath observer describes it this way:

Six days a week we wrestle with the world, wringing profit from the earth; on the Sabbath we especially care for the seed of eternity planted in the soul. The world has our hands, but our soul belongs to Someone Else...on the Sabbath we try to become attuned to holiness in time. It is a day on which we are called upon to share in what is eternal in time, to turn from the results of creation to the mystery of creation; from the world of creation to the creation of the world. (Abraham Joshua Heschel, *The Sabbath.* Farrar, Straus and Giroux. NY. 1951).

It becomes apparent that remembering the Sabbath is about much more than marking time in a week, though marking time is part of the music. Sabbath-observance is in the context of the larger symphony of life. The Creator-created relationship that is memorialized by the Sabbath is the pulse beat of *each* day. God says, "I gave them my Sabbaths, to be *a sign between them and Me*, that they might know that I am the Lord who sanctifies them... Hallow my Sabbaths, and they will be a sign between me and you, that you may know that I am the Lord your God" (Ezekiel 20:12, 20, *HCSB*, emphasis supplied).

God is identified as our Sanctifier. This means that God begins and finishes his pledge to make us holy and pure. This highlights again God's intentions. In time and eternity, He will sort out and remove the chaos that threatens. Another word stands out in this passage: "...that you may *know*..." Knowing speaks of intimacy and affection. There is nothing casual, fleeting, or haphazard in this relationship. This is not a cursory expunging of pain. The Sabbath relationship is about an abiding rest, one that endures through time.

Indeed, God gives more than a weekly 24-hour chunk of time so that we may know Him, though he gives us that too in a special way. God joins with us from First-day chaos to Seventh-day wholeness, integrating the fullness of heaven's graces into our personhood. We are never apart from Him, and He has given us His Sabbath as a definitive assurance that this is so.

We often start our prayers, "Dear Father in Heaven...," thereby claiming a relational dynamic. In the same way, our week may start with God-seeking faith and then progress throughout the week's ups and downs. We conclude our prayers with *Amen!* thereby declaring the authenticity of intentions and desires. (Translated, *amen* means "So be it!" "Let it be so!")

In the same way, we may end each week with a body-soul-spirit declaration that we fully accept God's authorship and ownership of us, and that we yield to His power and authority to save and heal us. We give him "breathing room" and He takes up residence in us just as He does within the Sabbath of His creation.

In the midst of chaos, this means that our swirling performance anxieties and feelings of inadequacy become more manageable. They find a place to land and are diffused. The adequacy of the Creator God in all circumstances is such that, if permitted, He will free the tumultuous heart from its turmoil, allowing the caregiver to be a truly living, non-anxious presence. I have found no other anchor point that works so well in turbulence.

The Sabbath guides and informs my heart as an expression of who God is as my Creator and Savior. Sabbath reminds me of God's capacity and desire to bring order out of chaos and provide rest and freedom from *all* illness for *all* humankind. It informs my attitude as I enter patients' rooms. God, not I, is the ultimate repairer of whatever may be wrong both within them and within me. When I remember that God is both Sovereign Most High and yet present in my being, I am able to remain more present to patients.

When I am tired, I am aware that I start to disengage, to lose my emotional availability. However, as I remember the Sabbath, I am brought back to the fulcrum of my being and given increased clarity and capacity for caring. Resting upon the sacred pivot point of grace, I can let go and let God do what God alone can do. In this sense, rather than me being a keeper of the Sabbath, the Sabbath becomes my keeper. It holds and sustains me. The Sabbath reminds me that when I desist from frenetic doing, God's being – the Infinite I AM – is doing what I cannot do. In the Sabbath, I experience God descending into human time, touching humanity, touching me, and restoring wellness where my efforts are futile. The Sabbath informs me about the One to whom I belong, my Creator. And it from this knowledge of restorative grace that I minister to His creation.

When God invited us to remember the Sabbath, His language indicated that true remembrance crosses all time zones and time lines. We are invited to make *each* conscious and unconscious moment an occasion for welcoming God's rest-giving-goodness within, allowing ourselves to ride His trajectory toward the sacred crescendo, that ultimate settling into the Sabbath fullness of God's righteousness – which is VERY good.

DE-STRESSING IN SEVEN BREATHS

Remembering the Sabbath can be thought of as a discipline of breathing, a venture between God and us. In the rush of each day, there may not be time to oxygenate in a favorite place, but there is a Sabbath breath that comes to us wherever we are, whatever the hour. As we open ourselves up and breathe prayers heavenward, we may increasingly experience rest in the midst of massive turbulence. The following are not unlike oxygen masks that fall from above when our flying carpet is being shredded:

1. **Affirm the Creator-created relationship**. Breathe out, "I can't fix this." Breathe in, "But, God, you can!" As we acknowledge our personal limitations and reliance for life on the Divine Presence, something starts to shift. Control passes outwardly. When we exhale, inhaling automatically follows! Self-opening allows a God-filling.

2. **Live life in the moment.** Breathe out, "Lord, I give you this day. Breathe in, "Give me your daily bread." Cherish each moment, acknowledging that all that pertains to life is a precious gift from our Maker. But, more than this, be aware that while God invites us to live within His eternal presence, His will is always in the context of the now. He told Moses, "Choose you *this* day whom you will serve." Tomorrow's Sabbath rest is a culmination of settling into God's abiding presence on *each* day that God gives. Living life in the moment is really about taking life in segments, one day at a time. We cannot breathe tomorrow's air today. Nor do we want to breathe yesterday's air for very long for it would become quite stale. Each day's breath is sufficient for the day.

3. **Anticipate God's timing.** Breathe out, "I give you my time!" Breathe in, "God, I accept your timing!" This is a matter of trusting in the processes of God's grace. In Psalm 1, the ancient chorister sings of what happens when one rests in the place where God

intends: "He is like a tree planted by rivers of water... He brings forth fruit *in its season*" (Psalm 1:3, *NIV*, emphasis supplied). Just as fruit drops into our hands when the right time comes, so also does God accomplish His purposes in all areas of our lives. Significantly, in the songster's original tongue, the nurturing river was really an irrigation canal. It was a stream directed specifically and intentionally to the tree from a bountiful source in order to nurture every stage of growth. The tree's task is to send down roots, anticipating that the Master Vintner will rejoice to see the results of time in His presence. God's time will yield a holy harvest.

4. **Expect valleys and mountains, shadows and sunshine.** Breathe out, "God, here I am." Breathe in, "God, meet me where I am." Our lives take our feet in many directions, encountering ebb and flow, a rising and falling, a moistening and a drying. In an era when many people viewed mountaintops as *the* place to meet the sacred, the psalmist cried out, "I lift my eyes to the hills. Where does my help come from?" The Creator responded to Him with assurances that holy help is available throughout *all* creation, including in low places. As God companions with us, we may have a heightened sense of His presence on one day and then experience a feeling of impoverishment on another. Yet, God's blessing may be found in both. As we ascend and descend, we may feel that it is "two steps forward, and one backward." Yet, we may be confident of this: God carries us unceasingly forward over both mountain passes and dizzying valley gullies. Atmospheric shifts may cause us stress, but God's breath is there.

5. **Make room for the new.** Breathe out, "God, I give you my brokenness." Breathe in, "God, make me whole." Behind my home is a sawdust sanctuary full of tools and projects. I retreat there to hammer, saw, drill, plane, chisel, sand, or simply ponder. Sometimes an accumulation of broken tools and unusable scraps muddle my pondering and projects. So, I periodically take inventory. Broken or unusable items are moved into a pile that I may look at and ponder for a while before hauling them away. In the same way, prayerful soul-searching tells when it is time for a trip to Heaven's Garbage Transfer Center. For any of us, unloading what no longer works may be painful, but it creates space and opportunity for more productive pondering and creativity. This might mean giving up cherished beliefs and

religious practices. Yet it opens the way for heaven's pure breath to enter and ride the highways of our being.

6. **Simplify what overwhelms.** Breathe out, "God, I give everything!" Breathe in, "Show me what matters most." Birth contractions surge through the body in excruciating waves. How does one endure? In the birthing process, is there not a time for labor and time for rest? Pain is often managed by focused, controlled breathing as the pain strikes. In between spasms of fire are pauses to regroup. Chunking down the process into segments allows joy to remain, especially when one's lover breathes alongside, helping to set the pace, all in anticipation of a sacred mystery, the emergence of a breathing, responsive expression of the Divine.

7. **Claim God's promises.** Breathe out, "All I am and hope to be I give to you." Breathe in, "All of you, I claim." As a child, oak trees surrounded my home. Acorns covered the ground each year tantalizing me with their inner meat. Stories of how First Nation's people ate them prompted me to take my pocketknife and skin a few for lunch one day. Never will I forget the taste of my first acorn. Bitter, disgusting, and repulsive! Little did I know that they first needed to undergo a long process of soaking, washing, and rinsing. Such is life! But even more, I was amazed to see that each acorn contained the essential elements of an oak tree in very tiny form – root, stem, and branches. I planted some of them and watched them grow. Like acorns in our hands, God's promises contain the fullness of life. When we apply our faith to them, we find rest in the shelter of an expanding mystery and sustenance from which bitterness has been removed.

THE WORLD IS SO EMPTY
IF ONE THINKS
ONLY OF MOUNTAINS, RIVERS AND CITIES.
BUT TO KNOW
SOMEONE WHO THINKS
AND FEELS WITH US,
AND WHO, THOUGH DISTANT,
IS CLOSE TO US IN SPIRIT,
THIS MAKES THE EARTH FOR US
AN INHABITED GARDEN.

Johann Wolfgang von Goethe

Chapter 2

HOLDING SPACE
FOR EVERYONE

RISING ABOVE TOXICITY

Sagebrush and rattlesnakes pepper the desert landscape in Washington State's Columbia Basin where I live. This is where the Columbia, Yakima, Snake, and Walla Walla Rivers converge on the way to the Pacific Ocean. Three cities – Richland, Pasco and Kennewick – bump against each other here on the rivers' embankments. It is indeed a place of abundance. Lots of sunshine, lots of heat, lots of cold! And lots of toxicity!

Environmentally aware inhabitants ask, how safe is the air we breathe? How healthy is the water we drink? These are not insignificant questions when one lives a one-eyed frog's hop, skip, and jump away from the waste products of nine decommissioned nuclear reactors, five former plutonium-processing plants, and residual crud from the production of 60,000 cold war nuclear bombs.

Fifty-three million gallons of high-level nuclear waste are stored underground nearby, much of which was buried utilizing inadequate technology. This is two-thirds of America's nuclear waste, and makes this region the most contaminated spot in the United States (http://en.wikipedia.org/wiki/Hanford_Site, retrieved August 31, 2012). This is my hospital's home turf. Can such an environment really deliver wellness to the 300,000 people who now live nearby?

My dad was a young soldier preparing for the invasion of Japan when Hanford was making history as part of the Federal Government's

Manhattan Project. Fat Boy, the nuclear bomb detonated over Nagasaki, Japan on November 6, 1945, carried plutonium from this area and effectively thinned Nagasaki's population by more than 60,000 inhabitants in an instant. Some say that Hanford's plutonium contributions possibly saved my father's life, ending the war before he was flung into battle. As a non-weapon-bearing conscientious objector and soldier-medic, Dad always felt conflicted by the success of Fat Boy. The loss of life saddened and angered him. Yet, he lived and I am glad.

While Dad was bivouacking in Hawaii en route to the Far East, the government started a small medical facility in Richland to support the burgeoning work force. During the war years, starting in 1943, America built the world's first full-scale plutonium processing plant on the banks of the Columbia River adjacent to Hanford, Washington, a sleepy farming town of 900 people. The nearby community of Richland mushroomed overnight from 250 people to more than 50,000 people in support of a secretive round-the-clock effort to end World War II quickly.

That first hospital opened in a rustic farmhouse. Inadequacies were immediately apparent. So, it was soon moved to a women's barracks. Soldiers and government workers – and their offspring – immediately overran this. Thus, by January 1944, the Army Corp of Engineers and the DuPont Corporation, a primary government contractor, started building a 55,000 square-foot Quonset hut complex.

Lieutenant Colonel Harry R. Kadlec, the Army Corp of Engineer's Chief Engineer and overseer of all major construction projects in the government town, was the first person to die in the new facility. Eight days after he suffered a fatal heart attack, Old Glory flew at half-mast overhead in his honor, and the new hospital was named after.

A decade later, Kadlec Hospital passed from government ownership and control to the Methodist Church, becoming one of only a few government-run hospitals to ever be privatized. In 1971, the hospital's Board of Directors turned it over to a new non-profit community-based corporation that renamed it Kadlec Medical Center.

Now known as Kadlec Regional Medical Center (KRMC), the hospital that once served only U.S. government workers, soldiers, and their dependents has become the leading medical referral center for a diverse populace in southeastern Washington State and northeastern Oregon.

Buildings that reflect the region's growth replaced the original military Quonset huts long ago (http://www.kadlec.org/krmc/about).

The hospital's latest addition towers over the city that has grown up where the village once was. The River Pavilion matches the height of the Federal Building several blocks away. While federal agencies monitor multiple entities involved in the cleanup of Hanford's radioactive wastelands, Kadlec receives those whose brokenness cries out for wellness in body, mind, and spirit. The landscape of the land and the landscape of the human soul both cry out for healing. Chaplains are part of this landscape. Their prayers are for the healing of the earth and all humankind.

High inside Kadlec Regional Medical Center's River Pavilion are two steel beams that are part of a sky bridge linking old and new parts of the hospital. On them are handwritten the names of many of the hospital's 2,400 employees. As the beams were raised into place by a giant crane, two chaplains' antiphonal voices echoed through the spring air. Here is what staff and community heard:

A PRAYER FOR THE SACRED IMPRINT

Lord, on these two beams in front of us we have placed the imprint of our hands, writing our names with indelible ink. We ask now that you permanently place the signature of your sacred blessings upon this structure.

Bless these beams of steel and all to which they are connected.

From its foundation depths to its crowning heights bless this building.

Bless these beams of steel and all who walk beneath.

Lord, from the tips of our toes to the top of our heads, bless us.

Bless these beams of steel and all the lives that are strengthened and supported by the care that they represent.

As these two beams of steel arise and settle into their resting places, hold them securely. In the same way, by your infinite wisdom, rivet

each heart to the hearts of others, making this hospital a safe place for people to work, rest and heal.

Bless these beams of steel as a reminder of what is real.

Lord, we desire that this skeleton of steel and concrete become a living entity, a vibrant organism containing a heart that is kind and good and true, and at the same time we ask that our own hearts of flesh might feel the autograph of your hand. Engrave your eternal love in all that is under, over, and around us.

Bless these beams of steel as symbols of infinite strength.

Lord, in their resting place high above the chaos of emotional, physical, and spiritual pain, may these steel beams, though out of sight, not be forgotten.

Bless these beams of steel that they may be a memorial of faith, hope, and love – the ties that keep us going.

Lord God Most High, bless these beams of steel and hold them in heavenly places.

Amen.

Surfing Currents
of Faith, Hope and Love

The overhead intercom shrills, "Code Blue, Orchard Pavilion, Room 327." I am in motion before the summons echoes through my pager. As I draw close, doctors, nurses, respiratory therapists and others overtake me and press through the door and start their interventions. I glance inside and see an emaciated, white-haired woman who looks to be in her 80s. However, my census sheet indicates that Amanda is in her late 50's. While the team does chest compressions and prepares to intubate Amanda, I confer with the hospital supervisor. Family has gone home for some rest after an all-nighter at the patient's bedside. So, I phone and urge them to return to the hospital "as quickly and safely as you can." Susie, a daughter, arrives first, dashing out of the elevator 10 minutes later. I position her at the entry to her mom's room where she can observe the team's efforts to revive and stabilize her mother. I stand alongside, steadying her. Our words are few. Then, we hear a shout, "We've got a pulse!" There are cheers, tears and smiles all around. Susie and I watch a while longer from the doorway, then I take her to a nearby family consultation room where she can phone and update family. Suddenly, we hear again overhead, "Code Blue, Orchard Pavilion, Room 327."

Powerful medications pour into Amanda. Already, the team has done chest compressions for over 40 minutes. Concerns for this fragile cancer patient now shift to her brain. Has she had an anoxic brain injury? It is certainly possible. Though Amanda now has a thready, irregular heartbeat, she is fully dependent on a breathing machine and powerful drugs. A doctor comes and tells us that Amanda does not have the resilience to recover. She cannot live long even with the strong medications and the ventilator. She will not regain the quality of life that she sought. Death is inevitable. He wonders, should we listen to what Amanda's body and spirit are saying, and allow her to die in comfort with no more rib-breaking chest compressions? Susie's grief is palpable, but she signals to the team to stop. They do so. The care team disperses as I escort Susie to her mother's bedside. As Susie clasps her mother's hand, I encourage her, "Speak whatever is in your heart. Trust that your mother's heart of hearts can hear you."

Our words are few as we wait at Amanda's bedside for other family members to arrive. The breathing machine has been taken away. Monitors have been turned off, silencing all bells and alarms. There is only the sound of shallow, sporadic breathing. Susie tells me about her family, worrying about how her nine-year-old identical twins will react to their beloved grandma's death. Susie tells me of her mother's faith in God and of her devotion to her grandchildren. Susie wants Carrie and Carmen to remember all the good times.

Quietly the door opens and two young faces peer tentatively around its edge. Their eyes fasten on Amanda, their grandmother. Carrie and Carmen have arrived. Susie and I gesture and invite them to enter. They enter hesitantly, pausing to stand at a distance. Fear and worry etch their faces.

I look at the two small girls whose eyes are now moving back and forth from their mother to me. Their mother is paralyzed with grief and is seemingly tongue-tied. Amanda breathes softly, like a minnow occasionally surfacing for sustenance. Looking at Carrie and Carmen, I speak, "Carrie,

Carmen, I'm Tom. You've not seen your Grandma like this before. Right now she can't respond to you with words. But, I think that she can hear you. It's okay to talk to her. It's okay to touch her. I think her heart of hearts knows that you are here and can hear you." They move closer and stand alongside their mother opposite me. They touch Amanda's arms, face and hands. Their tongues spill out currents of "I love you." This is indeed a much-loved grandma.

Tears flow too. Carrie and Carmen know that Grandma is dying. I feel hints of tears in the corners of my eyes as I listen to them and think of my own grandchildren. After a few minutes, the twins look up at me with smiles. Behind them, their mother mouths, "Thank you!"

"Carrie and Carmen, tell me about your grandmother. What did she like to do with you?"

"They look at each other and burst out laughing, "Cooking. Baking."

"So..." I ask, "What did you make together?"

Again, in unison, they giggle, "Cookies! Everything."

"So..." I say, "Who cleaned up?"

They look at each other and again erupt in stereo, "We did!" Then they get very quiet, look at their grandma and confess, "Actually, Grandma did. She always helped us."

Their memories fill the room. Looking at them, I say, "You know, don't you, that you will always have your Grandma's love? Do you know that your Grandma's Bible says, 'Love is forever?' You will always love your grandma." They nod and smile back at me. Amanda continues her shallow breathing, her breaths becoming further and further apart.

Periodically Carrie and Carmen punctuate their silence with questions, "Does she hurt?"

No, I say. "She is not hurting. She's surrounded by your love. That helps."

As the vigil continues I ask Carrie and Carmen, "Can you tell me a little more about your Grandma? Before she got sick, when you weren't all cooking and messing up the kitchen, what did she really, really like? Did she like to go places with you?"

Again, I hear stereophonic laughter, "Japanese!" When they see my puzzled face, Carmen and Carrie tell how their grandmother loved to take them to Japanese restaurants and Asian stores in search of Japanese curios. Japanese? Wow, I think. After 30 years of ministering in the Japanese language, do I know anything Japanese? Is there anything Japanese that I might give to these twins to help them remember their Grandma's love? At that moment, a nurse sticks her head in through the door to see if we need anything. I ask her to bring some paper and a "sharpie." Moments later she returns with a clipboard, some paper and several colorful pens.

I hold up the clipboard toward the girls and tell them, "I want to give you something to take home with you – something Japanese that will remind you of the good times you had with your grandmother."

As they watch, I put a sharpie to the paper and quickly draw the 13 strokes of the ancient squiggly pictograph for "Love." It is not on fine parchment and my calligraphy is rough, but it is Japanese. I point to the center of the character and explain, "These strokes right here represent the heart. The heart is where love comes from. Carmen and Carrie, I want to give each of you one of these pictures so that you will always remember how much you are loved." I prepare two sheets, writing a child's name across the top of each: "To Carmen" and "To Carrie."

I then write in blue ink across the bottom of each paper, "Love is forever!" Carmen and Carrie accept the papers as if they are receiving pure gold. In that instant, I am aware that something profoundly wonderful and mysterious has just happened within me. It has been many years since I daily wrote and spoke in the Japanese language. But, now 13 complex pen strokes have suddenly risen unbidden from the remote recesses of my memory for the sake of two grieving children. Deep grace has touched me. I've just experienced a reminder that lessons learned years ago in pain are never really lost, and that nothing is wasted if I continue listening.

Amanda's breathing continues for an inexplicably long time as more and more family gather. Carmen and Carrie greet each new arrival, holding and waving their calligraphic signs like celebratory flags. There is now no fear, no tentativeness. "See, look! Love is forever!" Stories fill the space. When the family has all arrived, Susie asks that I offer a prayer of relinquishment for Amanda. In those moments as we circle Amanda's bed and prayerfully ask God to receive and hold her, her breath escapes her body, returning to God who gave it. Yet, love continues on...and on...and on...

PRAYING WITH UN-GRIM REAPERS

Of course, not every person celebrates the presence of a chaplain. Early in my healthcare career, I responded to a Code Blue in our emergency department. While I waited for the patient's family members to arrive, someone walking down the corridor toward me saw my chaplain's badge and instantly fainted and collapsed on the floor. Despite what some might think, chaplains really are not grim reapers! In fact, I am usually very un-grim.

Now, to prevent panic attacks at first encounters, I sometimes flip my badge over until I can first introduce myself as a "hospital support person, here to help with your needs and wishes, whatever they might be." I then clearly identify myself as a chaplain. As a spiritual caregiver, I feel called to acknowledge the fullness of the human experience in all of its dimensions, affirming the realities of both pain and joy. It is a journey with one foot on the edge of a grave – my own and that of others – and the other foot solidly on hope. *Especially, I want to convey hope.* This is the theme of many of my prayers. What follows are prayers that I've offered when our hospital opened new healing spaces.

A PRAYER FOR A NEW MEDICAL TOWER

We dedicate this tower for restoring health where there is brokenness. May the joys and sorrows that are shared here create a community of hope!

We dedicate this pavilion for the healing of body, soul, and spirit. May its walls hold sacred the thoughts, feelings, and woundedness of all who enter.

We dedicate this place to listening for and honoring unspoken needs and wishes. May its roof provide a canopy for sheltering each person from the storms of despair!

We dedicate this tower for the upholding of human dignity. May its corridors take away haunting memories and bring refreshing, cleansing friendships!

We dedicate this pavilion to the outpouring of kindness. May its furnishings bear witness that comfort can be found in unfamiliar places!

We dedicate this place to the appreciation and implementation of all that is good and true. May its floors, doors, and corridors direct hearts toward wisdom!

We dedicate this pavilion as a threshold to all that transcends sickness and death. May its windows enable all to see farther and higher, to glimpse the sunrise coming with healing in its wings!

We dedicate the time and talents of those who serve here. May all feel treasured, nurtured, and empowered as agents of transformation and wellness!

We open both our hearts and this facility today in consecration to the service of humankind. May our offering today bring healing in its stream!

May heavenly kindness flow toward all who enter and depart from here, and in that current of love, may all know that this River Pavilion exists for the well-being of body, mind, heart, and spirit.

Lord, bless this River Pavilion now in the name of all that is healing and holy.

Amen!

A PRAYER FOR A NEW PEDIATRIC CENTER

Generosity allows creativity. When Don and Lori Watts' wheat ranch made them comfortably wealthy, their hearts turned toward the uncomfortable, particularly toward children and their parents. As a result, their generous donation jump-started the construction of a new state-of-the art pediatric center.

An interdisciplinary team of pediatric specialists crisscrossed America looking for innovative ideas to help make children feel cherished. The new pediatric unit is a high-tech marvel, skillfully combining the ambiance of an aquarium, petting zoo, and museum with the comfort of a family's living room. Every child's room has an individualized feel with floor mosaics and wall art depicting myriad quirky, absurd, and amazing creatures. Play areas perpetuate the aquatic theme with a climb-aboard boat and other stress-relieving nautical nonsense. Yet, it is a place devoted to serious treatments. These currents were captured in a prayer at ribbon-cutting time:

Almighty Healer and Compassionate Friend, when the seas of life threaten to overwhelm with waves of sickness, pain, and grief, in this place, send forth the currents of peace, hope, and relief.

When creatures of destruction intimidate our senses, in this place, send alongside messengers of compassion and healing.

When sorrow seems to saturate our world, in this place lift up each person's heart through any and all gloom into the Sunshine of Transcendence.

As children and their loved ones enter here, may their senses feel the undercurrents of enduring love! May they see every creature on the Center's walls, floors, and ceilings, and in the fish tanks as evidence of a Most Loving Heart, of a Creator Friend who brings laughter and hope with colorful caricatures of the absurd and the magnificent!

Light of Glory, shine into this place through every window.

Smile with favor upon each child, blessing every body – fingers, toes, feet, and nose – with tenderness, easing pain, knitting together that which is broken – into a new and glorious representation of Goodness. Bless not only the body, but also the spirit within.

Today as this ribbon is cut, opening this Pediatric Center, our spirit expands outward to receive heaven's favor and to commit ourselves to making this place a sanctuary where healing touches the whole person.

Light of the Endless Sky, as sea and sky meet here under this roof, open this planet to receive the light that shines outward from the windows of this fifth floor through gloomy days and during the night.

May the Messengers of the Deep and You, the Light of Endless Ages, You Who Are on High, converge in this place and surround each child with reminders of all that endures: faith, hope, and love – a faith that clings to what is true, hope that grasps tomorrow, and love that is as deep, wide, and full as the ocean.

In this moment, we claim the fullness of heaven's blessings for this Pediatrics Center.

Amen.

A Prayer for a New Acute Care Unit

Divine Caregiver of All the Earth,

Today as we cut this ribbon to open this new floor, we seek to cut through the non-essentials to those things that matter most. This is our heart's desire:

May this new Sixth Floor be a home-like sanctuary of wisdom and grace where people say, "I care," and truly mean it. Strengthen our capacity, O Lord, to love.

May what is seen and heard here on this unit invoke a spirit of thanksgiving for what has been and what will be.

May the earth-toned paint on walls remind of the touch of the Holy One upon human clay; May the airiness of the broad, bright landscapes that flood through windows infuse breath and life into the weary, and may hope not be dimmed when lights and machines are switched off!

In the shadows of painful choices, may none grieve alone as those who have no hope! Lord, grant eyesight that transports beyond the horizon into the Ultimate Healing Presence. Strengthen our capacity, O Lord, for thankfulness.

May this new Sixth Floor provide space for brokenness to be healed, especially the brokenness that lies beyond the touch of ointments, pills, and other treatments! Lord, touch deeply where forgiveness is needed.

May the colors of grace and the textures of compassion be buttressed by a resolve of steel to make things beautiful in every relationship! When a cure is not possible, may there yet be a healing within the heart. Strengthen our capacity, O Lord, to forgive and be forgiven.

So, Creator and Healer of Humankind, strengthen our capacity to truly care. As we cut though today's ribbon, we ask that you empower us to cut through the transitory things of this life to manage our lives and our caregiving on this sixth floor with love, gratitude, and grace. As we step forward in your presence, Lord, bring us to this Highest Level of Caring.

Amen.

A NOON BLESSING FOR A NEW MEDICAL BUILDING

As the sun reaches its zenith overhead, we pause to ask heaven's blessings upon our endeavors. We pray:

Almighty Architect of Hope, descend upon this site, touching our plans and dreams with your favor.

As the concrete foundations of this building are poured, spill out upon this ground your divine purpose – unshakable and solid, upholding our vision for healing.

As walls and roof are raised, lift up the hearts of the medical practitioners whose hopes are centered on the wellness of both individuals and our community.

As windows and doors and furnishings are placed, open wide our spirit to see and know what really matters.

As medical equipment is installed, may all who enter here be enthralled not by the newness of things and the freshness of paint, but by the freshness of hope and the anticipation of soul-wholeness even when a cure cannot be found.

Through the dust and debris of construction let there be freedom from the destructive forces of injury or accidents. Come alongside each worker, whatever his or her role, so that the body and soul of each is safe and secure.

Beloved Healer, make this place a Sanctuary of Transcendence for this community –

> *A place where discourse is not hoarse or coarse but civil,*
> *A place where hope supplants despair,*
> *A place where wellness is greater than death itself,*
> *A Sanctuary of Transcendence – a model of the Highest Level of Caring.*

Finally, Lord, for touching the mortal mortar of our lives with great grace, we give our gratitude.

Amen.

CLEANSING A TRAUMATIZED OPERATING UNIT

Sometimes doctors, nurses and other clinicians speak of heavily burdened places in the hospital where infants have died or where organs have been "harvested" for transplant after a tragic motor vehicle accident. Where deaths occur as a result of violence, whether self-inflicted or otherwise, it seems that grief permeates the pores of walls, floors and those who work there. It can be hard for staff to return to places of painful memories. One day, following the death of another battered infant, a surgeon cried out, "I hate this room!" This prompted a nurse to suggest that chaplains be called to come and cleanse the space. Her suggestion evolved into a decision to cleanse and bless each surgical suite with a voluntary prayer time.

Thus, early one morning all non-emergent surgeries were pushed back for a later start, and forty OR staff gathered with three chaplains in front of a nursing station. Here is how the cleansing time was scripted:

In the midst of the brokenness and blessedness of life, we pause for a short while this morning to renew this place and ourselves. From ancient times, olive oil has had special significance for it comes from olives that have been bruised, beaten, and crushed, bringing flavor to food, light to lanterns, and life to the world. It illuminates darkness and nurtures bodies. Its fragrance is not overpowering, but touches the senses as a gentle presence, bringing a message of tender caring. Representing the "wounded healer," the oil has sacred meaning, symbolizing both the healing influences of the Divine Spirit and of the healing arts. So, this morning we have brought olive oil, frankincense and myrrh, blended together according to a 3,000 year old recipe in a fragrant reminder of that which transcends suffering and death. This oil represents the consecration of our lives to bringing wellness to others. Join me now in a prayer for cleansing and renewal:

Beloved Guardian of our Minds, Hearts, and Bodies, in the spaces of our hearts and the rooms of this floor, we ask:

> That you surround us with your protective graces,
> That you cleanse away all that harms, hurts or destroys the well-
> being of patients, their families and staff,
> That you bring wholeness where there is brokenness.

Bless every space, every place.

In the spaces of our hearts and the rooms of this floor we implore that as we place your anointing oil above each door that you will mark each opening with the outpouring of your blessings upon the surgical team, giving to each person wisdom, compassion and skill and that you will remove all toxic and tainting influences.

Bless every space, every place.

In the spaces of our hearts and the rooms of this floor, we implore for:

> More serenity in the knowledge of what we can change,
> More tranquility in recognition that human brokenness
> is not forever because of the Infinite One,
> More confidence in the Divine mastery of the mystery of life!
> More assurances that our lives are held in
> holy compassionate hands.

Bless every space, every place.

In the spaces of our hearts and the rooms of this floor,

Where there has been death, let there be hope.
Where there has been sadness let there be gladness.
Where there has been brokenness let there be healing.

Bless everyone – surgeons, anesthesiologists, nurses, technicians – everyone!

We implore, Lord God, make all things new and light now in the freshness and power of your holy favor.

Hear this prayer. O Lord.

Amen.

At this juncture the three chaplains invited the OR's team to form a circle and extend their hands, palms upward.

You have chosen to bless others with your hands in the work you do. Now we want to bless your hands in recognition of the sacredness of what you do each day. This initial blessing is for the work you do personally. Please extend your hands outward with palms up to receive the holy presence. "With this oil, may your hands be strengthened and soothed that they may strengthen and soothe others."

Now clasp hands with each other, allowing the oil to flow from hand to hand. The mingled oil represents the serving community of which you are a part. This blessing is for the work that you do as a team. "Now may God bless all of your hands as they work together, that they may continue to be a blessing to others in the days ahead."

So, what is next? Each of you, lift the oil to your nostrils and savor its fragrance. Now, let us spread the oil throughout this floor, from corridor to corridor, from room to room. We invite you to transfer the oil with the touch of your hands to all the places that you feel need special healing. As you pass through or alongside doors or wherever, we invite you to each lift up the desires of your hearts in either audible or silent prayer, either privately or with a friend.

The Nightingale Lamp in the hands of our Perioperative Manager will lead the way. Natalie's lamp and our candles (battery powered) signify the pervasive presence of the Divine in all aspects of life, affirming that just as fire and light cleanse, so also does the Sacred One purify and illuminate the dark places of our lives.

Also, please know that you may pause at any time to obtain from the chaplains a replenishment of the oil in your hands. May the sacred oil impart its healing graces upon all that it touches, and may the Light of Heaven dispel all darkness now. Walk in peace!

Amen!

Praying at the Crossroads For a New Free-Standing Emergency Department

Today we stand at the a crossroads of Highway 395 and 19ᵗʰ Avenue. Roads converge. Roads intersect. This facility even has its own turn lane!

Over the past year, I have watched this facility rise from the ground to change the landscape of our community. Seeing the changes and contemplating today's opening ceremony, my thoughts have turned to an ancient wise man who viewed crossroads as a place of sacred choices. The prophet Jeremiah said, "This is what The Lord says, 'Stop at the crossroads and look around. Ask for the old, godly way and walk in it. Travel it's path, and you will find rest for your souls'" (Jer. 6:16, NLT).

So, we stop, we look, we ask the way, and we walk in it. Join me now this morning as we invoke the guiding hand and healing touch of the Most Holy upon all who pass by or enter Kadlec's new free-standing emergency department.

Lord of All Compassion and Power, help us to ask each day: What is right and good and transformative of pain, whether that pain be physical, mental, emotional or spiritual. At this crossroad, may your Sacred favor be the signal light that directs all toward wholeness.

Where disease intersects with life's fears, help us to find the answers that matter most. Provide the turn signals that direct toward wellness.

Lord, we ask that you fill this place with love and compassion. May the sacred medicine of compassion converge with knowledge and wisdom and then travel beyond these four corners throughout our community and to the four corners of our fractured planet. Let this be a healing place for humanity.

Lord, just as light penetrates this healing center through many windows, please let the transparency of our hearts intersect with kindness. Let our honesty never be cruelty. Let us do no harm. Help us to be good and do good. Let us heal like the light shining in darkness.

Lord, begin with us. Where our personal and institutional weaknesses and failures intersect with people's overwhelming needs, transform us that we may be transformative healers for all who come to us seeking respite from their troubles. Pour the joy of service into us, bringing within us a convergence of our passions, skills and sense of calling. May this happen in such a way that all experience rest from afflictions, anxieties and pain.

May this intersection pull together people whose needs coincide with what this facility and this staff have to offer. Help us to succeed in the purposes for which we are here. Like the rooflines of the building that stands behind us, Lord, point our goals upward and outward. Direct us toward that which transcends the pain of our mortality.

Finally, Lord, we want to voice our gratitude for those men and women whose vision, talents, and commitment have converged on this site to transform not only the landscape of this intersection of highway 395 and 19th Avenue, but also transform lives in a quest for wholeness. We give thanks for visionary leaders, planners, developers, construction workers and all who labor on behalf of those who come to this crossroad.

As scissors now intersect with this ribbon in this morning's ribbon-cutting ceremony, we ask that your heart of perfect love will intersect with ours, filling our hearts with all of your blessings.

Amen.

DISRUPTING THE EQUILIBRIUM

It is sometimes said that the longest and most difficult road in the world is the pathway between the head and the heart. Some people struggle to get in touch with their emotions while others marinate in them. Some people know their own minds, but can't name the awe that they feel when they see a gorgeous sunrise or sunset. Others are like Charlie, our little Yorkie dog who sometimes pants and sneezes at moths, envisioning them as tasty morsels. Like Charlie, they sneeze at new thoughts, but are always ready for a laugh or a cry. Saying "Bless you!" to them doesn't change these wheezing geezers any more than explaining the nutritional value of cheerios inspires Charlie.

In this regard, rituals may aid transformation. There are at least two types of rituals. First, there are rituals associated with "the old time religion," ones that quickly evoke a flood of memory associations. An example of this is the Holy Eucharist as shared within the Catholic Church and many Protestant traditions. Familiar words and movements evoke a sense of timelessness. Familiarity re-anchors a person who is grappling for something that has been lost. The second type of ritual breaks from the familiar, and thereby disrupts the equilibrium. The unfamiliar creates a disquiet that tickles the mind and heart to adventure in new directions. Either type of ritual causes a type of internal shift – either shifting a person from temporary chaos back to groundedness, or shifting a person from stuckness toward disequilibrium and thence toward internal resolution.

Here is a tickling kind of hand blessing, spoken to caregivers who came to the hospital's chapel expecting their hands to be anointed with familiar oil:

A Hand-blessing Ritual:
"You are like a feather!"

A feather has softness, gentleness and tenderness.

Your gentleness touches mysteriously and lightly, stirring breezes of goodness as you come alongside patients and their families.

A feather has great strength. Your presence alongside patients and family members imparts power to journey with hope.

A feather has many facets. Like a feather with a strong spine and multiple interlocking, interconnected pieces, you hold together in community people whose lives are buffeted by nasty storms.

You are conveyers of strength, life and courage.

As this feather touches your hands today, may you know that your hands equip others for flights of the soul!

May this feather's touch give wings to your heart and feet as you walk this hospital's hallways imparting strength to the bodies, minds and spirits of patients and their families. And may you know that no feather falls to the ground without being seen and known in heaven. You are precious and appreciated.

Amen.

A BLESSING OF PRAYER SHAWLS: THE FABRIC CLOSET

Well-crafted rituals engage mind, body and spirit, creating pathways from the mentally mundane to sacred possibilities by utilizing sensory triggers. While the mind recognizes something as common, our senses may move the heart to exclaim, Wow! The following ritual utilizes elements of guided imagery to reconnect persons with important aspects of their personhood.

Imagine for a moment: a place in which you feel whole.
> *As this shawl surrounds you, may it soothe you. May it enfold you like a gentle hand, caressing you tenderly.*

Imagine for a moment: a place where you do not feel alone.
> *As this shawl enfolds you, may you feel always close to the Holy One, finding rest in this place for your weariness; may it wrap around you like a heavenly hug, reminding you that you are precious to God; may it also become a pillow for you, a place to dream about new realities.*

Imagine for a moment: a place where tears are wiped away and there is no more sorrow, grief or despair.
> *As you close yourself within this fabric closet, may you breathe in the fragrance of heaven; may you know that the Holy One is very near to comfort and cheer, to remove all fear and to wipe away every tear.*

Imagine for a moment: You are yet a child nestled on your parent's lap.

Like a child at bedtime and a child awakening in the morning, may this shawl be a place to connect with all that is precious, pure and lovely.

Now imagine for a moment. You are a grown-up child.

As a child of the Holy One, may you experience your shawl as a constant reminder of where you came from and that to which you are called; may you, yourself, emerge from your fabric closet to be a shawl of blessing for all those whose lives you touch.

May you and your shawl be blessed by the Holy One today!

Colliding with Grace

As I scan the corridors of the Intensive Care Unit, I notice a frail-looking man leaning forward against the wall, touching it with his forehead. His body is trembling. I do not see his face but I recognize that he is sobbing. He stands by the entrance to a patient's room with his hands gripping a wall-mounted hand-sanitizing container. I do not want to startle him. So I approach cautiously. Gently, lightly, I touch his shoulder as I speak. "Hi, I'm Tom, part of the hospital's support staff. I want to respect your space and your needs, but I am wondering if..."

The man turns fully toward me as tears stream down his face. I feel his forearms aligning with my own as his hands wrap around my elbows. His grip is surprisingly strong as his body's weight settles into me. He lifts his head to look in my face, and in that instant I am struck by this stranger's uncanny resemblance to my own aging father. "She's dying," he sobs, referring to his wife. We continue to hold onto one another. In the ensuing silence, I am aware that this man's tears hold the memories of many years. I ask him his name.

"Bob," he says. I feel a visceral jolt. This is my father's name. I then ask, "Tell me, what does your wife like to be called?"

"Betty," he responds. This is my mother's name. I feel tears lurking at the edges of my eyes and a lump forming in my throat.

Mom and Dad are currently navigating through the jungles of dementia and bodily decline. Time is no longer just marching on, it is moving at jet-speed, leaving contrails of grief. With my parent's advancing age, I feel my own mortality, knowing that I may become, as they are, dependent on others for help with the activities of daily living. These are painful thoughts. With every fiber of my being, I want to cherish each day, hour, and minute. I am continuously aware of how fragile my existence is. So, I choose to live the lessons about hanging on and letting go that Mom and Dad have taught me. Hanging onto faith, hope and love, I let go.

My new friend Bob asks that I come and pray with Betty. We sanitize our hands and enter Betty's room and stand alongside her, Bob on one side of her bed and I on the other. We each take one of her hands as I pray, "God, thank you for all the memories that Bob and Betty share. Hold them both now in your arms that they may feel your love and grace. Sustain them with your healing hands and in your time, reunite them in that place where there will be no more good-byes, no more tears, no more sorrow or death." Lightly I touch Betty's forehead. "Now may the good Lord bless you and keep you. May the Lord smile upon you and give you his peace and rest, now and always. Amen."

As I depart, Bob smiles like a kind and loving dad toward me. I have received his blessing.

LEAVING A LEGACY OF TORN FABRIC

My sister has called to tell me that Dad has stopped eating. He barely and rarely talks now. We see that he is redirecting his energy toward letting go of life in this world. It's been quite a journey. I've watched his years of servanthood, how he's tended family needs, how he's mowed the lawn at church, how he's wrestled to know his own worth after not following in the footsteps of his father and grandfather who were highly regarded ministers. My heart celebrates his amazing processes of personal growth. This once wiry, strong-legged man has lived to the max, fighting personal demons to climb tall mountains and gaze at possibilities both nearby and over the next mountain range. He has lived a life of servanthood, no less impactful than that of his parents and grandparents. As he prepares for rest in God's presence, savoring sustenance that is not visible, I celebrate him.

I remember... Yes, indeed I remember a Sabbath afternoon walk with my Dad through a nearby field. His church-going necktie and jacket were gone. However, he still wore new suit slacks. We came to a barbed wire fence with no gate. Dad promptly paced away from the fence to show us the way over. With a hop, skip, and flying leap, Dad propelled himself into the air and landed upright on the other side. Awed by Dad's agility, my mom and siblings gazed at him and then at what he left behind on the barbed wire – a piece of fabric from the bottom of his suit trousers. Mom's agitated comment was, "Ohhh! Bob!"

Each day I encounter hospital employees and volunteers who lean into life, leaping and leaving in their wake something that stirs laughter, hope and joy. I am often asked to join with them for meals and special occasions. Of course, the cost of a meal is often a prayer. Here are some prayers that we've shared:

A Breakfast Blessing for Volunteers

Lord God, today we pause to celebrate the marvelous contributions of Kadlec's volunteers. For their sacrifices of time and resources, we give thanks. For their kindness toward staff, patients and families, we give thanks.

Through the aches and pains of life they keep going on and on and on, making life more manageable for our staff, patients and families. For this we give thanks.

They are always here, Lord, touching our lives with compassion and dedication. Though they work without pay, they do not stop. Pay them, Lord, out of the abundance of heaven's treasure house. May they know today that they are loved and appreciated! Reward them with the affirmation of your presence.

Give to each freedom from anxiety about the future. Give them joy in the knowledge that their efforts are making this world a kinder place. Give them peace in their hearts, assuring them that you hold each one in your hands in all that they do.

Now give to each a hearty appetite to enjoy all of your bountiful blessings. Bless the food now that we are about to eat.

Amen.

THICK LENSES, BRITTLE BONES AND FALSE TEETH

Beloved Giver of All Good Gifts, we turn our hearts and minds toward you now in gratitude for the abundance of your tender mercies toward us.

For waking us up in the morning; for touching our vision with the beauty of a new sunrise – even as we see through thick lenses; for filling our mouths with food that nourishes; for teeth, whether real or false, that can chew and enjoy your blessings; for filling our hands with tasks that bring pleasure to others and to you; for hands that touch and inspire life even while bones are brittle and hurting; for filling our hearts with the spirit of renewal and hope; for a pulse that is paced by you, the Heavenly Pacemaker; for all this, we pause to say, Thank you!

So, keep our hearts beating today, Lord, with the impulses of your love and grace!

For those senior members whose bodily aches and pains are cramping their style today I ask that you reach out and hold them where they are. Give them strength.

For those who are more youthful and newer to the joys of volunteerism, I beseech you: Launch them into the deep and sustain them. Give them wisdom and inspiration.

Now may all the hours that are volunteered here by this angelic group of Kadlec people be received into your heart as an expression of all that is good and holy and forever enduring!

We pray this now with full hearts in anticipation of full stomachs.

Amen.

SIXTY YEARS OF WHEELING, DEALING AND HEALING

O Divine One, Patron of Volunteers, some people toil because they have to, in order to put food on the table; to pay bills; to fill time until the workday is done. They sweat, grunt and groan for a paycheck, for accolades, for survival, for money to escape the drudgery of life with vacations, toys and exotic escapades.

But, Lord, those who are here tonight are different. They toil not because they have to...but because they WANT to. They want to help the broken and hurting to find hope and the power to cope; to make a difference by being different, by giving rather than taking. For them, O Lord, we give thanks.

Sixty years of volunteerism. Sixty years! Countless hours of smiling, greeting, wheeling, delivering, stitching, sorting, filing; repeated days of getting out of bed to once more fill a desk, fill an envelope, fill and push a wheel chair, and fill lives with hope where there is despair; unending service to Kadlec day after day, year after year, making a difference, not just to the hospital's bottom line, but especially within the lives of our patients, their families and staff.

Some, Lord, are no longer with us, having parted from this life. We remember them and ask that you will hold each to your heart tonight that each may know the heartfelt gratitude of the Universe.

For all our Volunteers, Lord, Yes, we give thanks.

Tonight, as representatives and recipients of 60 years of volunteerism, we shall mingle, socialize, and partake of good food. As we eat now, may every volunteer know the fullness of your Divine pleasure!

Amen.

An Anthem of Hope for Veteran Employees

Join me in gratitude now for those whom we honor tonight at this year's Recognition Banquet. May the words, thoughts, and desires of our hearts rise up together to give thanks for those who serve at our hospital – especially for those whose names will be read aloud this evening! Hear now the anthem of hope that we hold for one another:

We hope that each person knows that his or her presence at Kadlec matters. May all know that every year, every day, every hour, and every minute of service makes a difference in the lives of patients, family members and co-workers.

We hope that in the ebb and flow of life no one is invisible, forgotten, or overlooked. May we see tonight how dearly and how clearly each person is valued!

We hope that everyone from fresh-faced fledglings to grizzled veterans will find common cause in Kadlec's Highest Level of Care – competent, compassionate care that reaches beyond just the treatment of sickness to the treatment of persons – the healing of the whole person. May all who are here tonight find that the yearnings of the heart are met in the relationships that we cherish in the hospital and in our homes! May love and peace prevail in the entire world!

We hope that the food and the beverages that we are about to consume now will satisfy our palates and fill the nooks and crannies of our hunger. May our eating, drinking, and socializing tonight provide a vision of a healed world in which all are comfortably full, all are at peace, and all are well.

May these hopes be fulfilled in all who are here tonight!

Amen!

A PRAYER FOR HOLIDAY BLESSINGS

During this holiday season, even while there is significant global unrest, we pause for a while from our sometimes painful work to celebrate the commitment and sacrifices of coworkers. Join me in a prayer of gratitude.

Lord, as we eat here tonight, while we play tonight, we give thanks.

When we greet old friends and smile at new ones, we give thanks, and when we think of all that has come into our lives and all that has gone out of our lives during this past year, we wonder at how quickly time has passed, and we give thanks that we can slow down and relax for a while.

As we pause in this place, we invite the Holy Presence to surround us.

When we think of those employees who are honored tonight for their dedicated service, we give thanks. Lord, join us in our celebration. And be also with those who may not feel like celebrating. As the World struggles to find peace and wholeness during this season, be present to those who are apart from us and who may be in harm's way. Wrap your arms around our colleagues, patients, families and friends, and affirm your love, power and presence.

Now, may the fullness of our stomachs and the joy in our hearts tonight reflect the abundance of your gifts!

Amen.

CELEBRATING THE SPIRIT OF THE ROARING TWENTIES

For the opportunity to step into the spirit of the Roaring Twenties we are grateful tonight. Like those who had just fought the war to end all wars back in the last century, we want to kick up our heels and celebrate a new world with laughter, music, and the abundance of good food. Lord, join us in this celebration.

Like those who fought valiantly in trenches and bunkers for goodness's sake and returned home, leaving friends behind, we too want to engage fully in the dance of life. Lord, may your restorative Spirit be upon us.

Like those who know that abundance can quickly recede resulting in depression and despair, we proclaim our gratitude for what is ours – the prosperity of freedom and friendships, and of meaningful employment. Lord, we thank you for giving us so much.

So, tonight, we accept this time together as a lull from the stressors that are a part of every generation.

Finally, Lord, bless us who have so much.
    And bless those who have so little.

Bless those of us who are warm and safe.
    And bless those who are unsheltered, cold, and despairing.

May heaven's healing powers fill the earth with a peace and love that transcends seasons! May all brokenness be turned into joy!

Amen.

RENEWAL WITHIN DEATH'S SKIN

A glass jar sits on a glass plate on a mahogany table in the Chapel. Light from a nearby window filters through, highlighting the jar's contents. Hundreds of glass teardrops rest within the jar and upon the plate where the jar rests. A small sign says, "Long ago an ancient poet said to God, 'You keep track of all my sorrows. You have collected all my tears in your bottle'" (Psalm 56:8, *NLT*). The script invites Chapel visitors to take a teardrop from the plate and keep it as a reminder of a personal grief or loss, and then to take another and place it with a prayer into the vessel in memory of a special relationship. The memorial to tears is thus an expression of community. The fellowship of tears is not small. Nor is the God who holds the vessel.

Picture God in this moment. When we cry, the Holy One does not hold out to us a tissue box to say, "Stop crying," but instead offers a jar, giving permission to let our grief spill out. How strong must God be to hear and hold the sobbing heartache of humankind! How does He hurt as His hands receive our wordless yearnings? I visualize God bowed down over the vessel. Sacred tears fall, joining, mingling and merging with ours to form a mobile prism of grace. A river runs through this jar, touching the shores of all humankind. This is the community of the Sacred.

In the ancient language, the jar is actually a wineskin. The hide of a slain sheep stretches to hold the harvest gold of a Master Wine-maker. The Sacrificed One holds death, redeeming it so that it contains and conveys a sacred covenant. Into the water and the wine of heartache, the Vintner infuses ingredients that are mysterious and real. I wonder: how big is the sacrificial wineskin that it can hold the tears of all humankind and at the same time hold the fullness of God's own pain?

Teardrops fall from heaven onto my spilled-out-heart. I am not tossed out or ignored. God is with me. I am not alone. In this place of tears there is a holiness that is vaster than this earth's ocean shores can contain. I feel it. As I wander hospital corridors, I experience the flood stream of Sacred Community.

Heeding an Old Fart's Tears

Jake was a curmudgeonly old geezer who was devoted to Bethulia, his apple-dumpling wife of sixty years. He always had a word or two for me as I rounded on the Intensive Care Unit where his wife was recovering from an incapacitating stroke. His countenance ebbed and flowed with hope, directly related to how she responded to medical treatment. Her prognosis was not good.

"How is she today?" I'd ask on Monday. "Better," he'd say.

"Not so good," he'd say on Tuesday.

"Same as always. Stubborn," he'd say on Wednesday.

Three weeks of ebb and flow with little progress. Then one day, I meet him near the entrance to The Chapel. He's headed from The Chapel to the Cafeteria. He gestures for me to stop. He wants to talk. His face is somber.

"Chaplain," he says. "I want you to know how much I appreciate your Memorial to Tears in The Chapel. Do you know I got a handful of those glass teardrops from the table and have shared them with my kids, and friends? Some of them have been across the country several times now. Those teardrops are holding us together!"

"That's wonderful!" I respond. "Let me know if you need some more."

"Actually, I wanted to tell you that I had to get another one," Jake says. "Yesterday I reached into my pocket to grab my teardrop and pray. You see, I rub it between my fingers when I pray. It helps me remember. But, yesterday it disappeared."

"Oh, I'm sorry. Do you know what happened?"

"Actually, I've got this ritual in the mornings. When I get dressed, I put Bethulia's teardrop in my pocket to help me remember…"

"Oh, that's good…great idea!"

"Actually, yes…I put it in my right pocket. And I put my daily pill – just one – in my other pocket. I take my medicine later in the day."

76

"Oh, what a great plan! Sounds like a good system!"

"Well, actually, yesterday I was walking down the hallway here and was feeling stressed about Bethulia. So, I stuck my hand in my pocket to retrieve the little teardrop to pray. But it wasn't there."

"Oh, I'm sorry. It sounds like that was stressful for you."

"Well, actually, I then reached into my other pocket," Jake explained. "No teardrop. But, my pill was still there!"

"Sooooo? You swallowed the…?"

"Yep!"

Long pause as I ask, "Sooooo? How is that for you?"

"Well, actually," he says. "This too shall pass!"

THE LIGAMENTS OF COMMUNITY

Like ligaments on bones, prayer has a capacity to join people together in ways that enable meaningful movement – even a dance toward joy. There is a fiber that runs through us that yearns for belonging and connectedness. We were designed to be in community. Yet, modern society pulls at our priorities to fragment us both individually and bodily. We too often become stretched and *str-r-r-e-e-tched* and *str-r-r-r-r-r-e-e-e-e-etched* beyond our capacity to enjoy the relationships that the Creator intended.

Loneliness is pandemic today even though we have marvelous means to transport people, voices and thoughts across great distances in ways unimaginable to our ancestors. Internet and satellite signals that encircle the globe fail to hug hearts with assurances that we are not alone. Ease of transportation does not fully ease the congestion of lonely angst. This fragmentation goes against humankind's innate design. Holy Writings indicate that God infused people with a core need and capacity to be in companionship with others. There is a groove that runs through our hearts directing us toward a kind of wholeness that cannot be experienced in isolation.

PUSHING THE RAILINGS

Robbie, age 81, had been in the hospital for over three weeks, recovering from open-heart surgery, complicated by a subsequent stroke. As I approach Robbie's room I am aware that love is a complex experience that contains both agony and joy. Upon entering, I see Robbie resting on his bed with his back and head elevated. Clara, his wife of 55 years stands beside him, her hands on his shoulders, rubbing his muscles. Robbie's face is expressionless, his eyes are unfocussed, and spittle dribbles down his chin. I observe that Robbie is inclining toward the edge of his bed. Were it not for stainless steel rails, he might topple over the side. Clara's face is somber. She smiles a tired smile as she sees me enter.

"Good morning, Clara," I greet her. "I'm wondering how you are this morning."

"Not so good," she says. "He's had a setback."

We step away from the bedside toward the entryway where we can still watch Robbie. I wonder whether he can hear us as we talk. "What are the doctors telling you?" I ask.

"It's not good. They say he may never make it home. It probably won't get better than this," she says, gesturing toward the bed. Tears spill from her eyes. "Look at him," she continues. He wouldn't want to live like this. Right now I don't know if he's even aware of us."

Clara moves back toward the bed and addresses her husband, "Robbie, remember the chaplain? Tom's here."

I greet him now, "Robbie, good morning," then catch myself wondering how it could possibly be "good." I notice now that Robbie's eyes wander. "I wanted to see you this morning; I've been thinking about you, wondering how you're doing." I notice that Robbie's upper body is pressing hard against the railing. I wonder how aware he is of his vulnerability. Does he realize how close he is to the edge of his bed and to the end of his life?

Clara notices Robbie's pressure against the bed railing, and pushes against his shoulder, trying to reposition him. "Robbie, Robbie! Are you okay? I don't want you to fall out!" Her frail strength is overwhelmed as more tears fall.

I speak again. "Robbie, Clara has been here every day. You know how amazing she is, don't you! She's never been far away. Fifty-five years together! Wow! That's a lot of memory-making!" I notice that Robbie's head and shoulders are now pressing even harder into Clara's hands as she continues her attempts to lift and push him toward the center of his bed. His body is resistant. His face with its drooling mouth shifts toward her, eyes still wandering.

Clara cries out, "Oh, Robbie, what am I going to do? Please! I don't want you to fall." In these words, I hear, "I don't want you to die!" Her age-spotted hands shove weakly against Robbie's shoulder, grappling to move him away from the railing that is flexing now. I am confident that it will not break, but I am not so sure about Clara.

A thought strikes me suddenly as I watch. "Robbie, are you trying to tell Clara something?"

Looking at Clara, I say, "Clara, I think Robbie's trying to tell you something!" We both pause to study Robbie.

Then, I say to Robbie, "Are you trying to say to Clara that you want to cuddle, that you want to snuggle?"

Instantly, Robbie's until-now expressionless face twists into a lopsided grin, his mouth laughing around his breathing tube. One eye focuses firmly on Clara and he nods his head decisively up and down.

"Well! Clara, it looks to me like Robbie is saying, 'I love you!'"

Robbie shifts his face toward me. He's grinning – lopsided still. His mouth is speechless. His eyes lock on mine, and suddenly he winks at me! It is an unequivocal, intentional wink. I am aware of deep emotions within me. I've just received an incredible, priceless gift. I am joyfully convicted that suffering cannot conquer love.

"Clara," I say. "No doubt about it! Robbie is saying to you, 'I love you!'"

Clara is laughing, crying, joyous, and momentarily speechless. Then she cries out, "I love you too!"

I recognize within me a deep need to NOT break their communion with my continued presence. I look at both of them, smile and step away, mouthing my silent farewell, "God bless you both!"

As I exit, I pull the privacy curtain closed behind me. My last sight of them is of their faces pressed together in a deep silent conversation.

WHEN CANYONS DIVIDE

Today, we often hear political pontificators and media pundits talk about a "gap" between people. Society splits itself into us-versus-them groupings of supposedly like-minded people. Whether the space between is called a small gap, a deep gulf or the Great Abyss, the reality is that people hurt when they are divided. They hurt themselves, they hurt others, and they miss the beauty of wholeness.

Imagine yourself walking along a sun-drenched beach in Hawaii. If you pause for a moment, you might find a deep-green, low-lying shrub spreading its branches toward the crashing waves, toward the sky and toward inland mountains. Bend down and look closely among the twisting branches and you will see an elegant white flower that is known as the ocean *naupaka*. Each cluster of white petals forms half of a circle; every blossom is shaped like a five-fingered single hand reaching out in supplication for an absent member.

Amazingly, we can find the ocean *naupaka's* perfect counterpart on distant mountain summits. The mountain version has a blossom that is the mirror image of the ocean *naupaka*. When the mountain *naupaka* blossom is held alongside that of the ocean *naupaka* the singular beauty of each is exceeded by the composite splendor of wholeness. Each completes the other. Held flat and open alongside one another they form a perfect bowl prepared to receive rainbow blessings. Held palm to palm, they gratefully affirm the power of an exquisite God.

In ancient island legends, the ocean and mountain *naupaka* blossoms represent lovers tragically separated by the difficulties of life. Yet there is hope. In the hands of the Transcendent One they are brought together. Extraordinary help is available to carry us across the gullies and canyons of broken relationships. Holy Writings indicate that God's hands stretch out relentlessly bringing wholeness where there is brokenness.

THE MOST SIGNIFICANT OTHER

Long ago, Daniel, a great sage of the Israelites, became distraught when he saw a vision in the night of his community being trampled underfoot by a terrifying and extremely strong enemy. He saw his people crushed, mangled and devoured by evil. And his heart cried out for relief.

Persistence paid off. "I kept looking until thrones were set up, and the Ancient of Days took his seat; His vesture was like white snow, and His hair like pure wool...Thousands upon thousands were attending Him, and myriads were standing before Him; the court sat, and the books were opened" (Daniel 7:9, 10, *NASB*).

Daniel's vision of the Holy One coming to judge and heal humanity touches my imagination. Why does God depict himself as old? Why is God's hair pure white? Certainly a God who is from everlasting to everlasting is always young. Why then the snowy white hair?

It is an indicator, I believe, of the Holy One's solidarity with all who have experienced the trauma of loss and grief. God is in community with us. More than a crown of silver and gold, white hair signifies a superlative kind of authority. It speaks of an authority that comes from a very personal painful journey. Indeed, God has direct, intimate knowledge and understanding of what it means to be crushed and trampled underfoot by evil. Every white hair on God's head tells of painful moments in God's eternity. This is the Sacred Friend who arises to resolve the chaos of the human condition!

Daniel writes, "I kept looking in the night visions, and behold with the clouds of heaven One like a Son of Man was coming and He came up to the Ancient of Days and was presented before Him. And to Him was given dominion, glory, and a kingdom that all the peoples, nations, and men of every language might serve him...And His kingdom will never be destroyed" (Daniel 7:11, 12, *NASB*).

Solidarity. Community. Oneness in a precious hope. On the sixth day of Creation Week, God (singular) said, "Let *us* make man in *our* image..." (Genesis 1:26, *KJV*). The One God spoke of a plural dynamic that exists within the Sacred. God is *never* outside of community. And community is always in God. Herein is a mystery and challenge. How do we live in such a way that our ways of being and doing reflect our origins and our destiny?

When Rubbed the Wrong Way

Somewhere in the night between His last meal and being nailed to a cross, Jesus, who often referred to Himself as the Son of Man, told His final story. As His betrayal and death approached, Jesus presented His Last Will and Testament to His disciples in a parable. He closed that message by saying, "I have told you this so that my joy may be in you and *that your joy may be complete*" (John 15:11, *HCSB*, emphasis supplied). Can there be anything more desirous or meaningful than claiming this promised inheritance?

So, what is Christ's last story? It is a story of community. "I am the true vine, and my Father is the gardener...Remain in me, and I will remain in you...As the Father has loved me, so I have loved you. Remain in my love" (John 15:1-4, 9, 10, *NCV*).

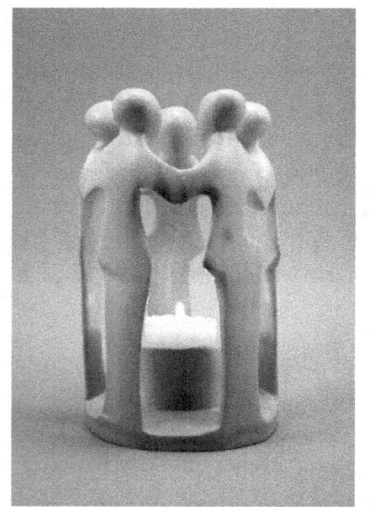

The story in its entirety portrays God as a vinedresser who takes vines that are non-productive and grafts them into a new Life Source that they may be energized and transformed. In other words, He connects us where we need to be connected, cleans away the muck into which we've fallen, lifts us up toward the light, and energizes us. He prunes us, protects us, and heals us from decay. It is a story of relentless healing mercy in all manner of relational dynamics. It is transformative.

There was a time in my life when I experienced the painful loss of a spouse. One day I was curled in a fetal position sobbing out my heartache to God with the only words that I could utter, "God! Have mercy!" Exhausted, I lay there in despair. Then I heard within my spirit a song from my childhood. "Jesus loves me this I know... Little ones to Him belong... We are weak but He is strong." Like gentle arms those words hugged and held me as I moved forward out of depression into a journey of hope.

Truly there is security and safety in this relationship. The Savior says, "Indeed I have called you friends." It is a companionship so deep that it is sealed with the Lord's own lifeblood. He says, "You did not choose me, but I chose you and appointed you that you go and bear fruit that will last" (John 15:16, *HCSB*).

Who has ever opened a fortune cookie and found life forever changed by its inner message? Such has been my experience. Bonnie is a beautiful woman both on the outside and the inside. We met long ago as young adults and then served in ministry on opposite sides of the world. After we each tasted the bitterness of loss, we met once again as middle-aged single parents in the presence of mutual friends. That encounter led to numerous exchanges of emails (more than 5,000 single-spaced pages) between my parsonage in Hawaii and her domicile in Oregon. Our friendship grew.

Then came the day that I flew to the Mainland to spend a week with her. Her warm heart and lips welcomed me. For the next week, she plied me with chocolate kisses and fortune cookies out of a bottomless bag as we drove around the Pacific Northwest visiting family and friends. Each hollow cookie contained a tantalizing, personalized message from her: "Tom, I am glad you are here!" "Tom, you are a good person." "Tom, I trust you." "Tom, I'm falling for you!" They were exclamation marks upon my emotions. How could I not love this woman!

By then I knew that I would ask her to marry me, if only I could find the right time, place, and words. Would she say, Yes? My shoes were on and I was headed out the door for church with her from my parents' home, when I jokingly (and quite seriously) said, "When we get to church this morning, what would you think if I signed the guest book 'Tom Becraft and Bonnie, his bride-to-be'?"

She looked at me and said, "Hold that thought!" as she disappeared back into Mom and Dad's guest room. She reappeared moments later and held out to me an elegant bag topped with puffy white paper. As I removed the tissue, I saw a pair of whimsical black socks embroidered with red hearts. Wow! I thought. Certainly my parishioners will smile when my pant legs rise up. No embarrassment! I will wear them with joy, thinking of Bonnie.

Then I noticed something more. Beneath the socks was a perfectly packaged, flawless fortune cookie, securely sealed in its original cellophane wrapper. After a week of tantalizing fortune cookie notes I wondered how many more surprises Bonnie could give me. This time, she spun my mind, heart and soul into highest orbit with her message: "Tom, I love you. Will you marry me?"

Being chosen is totally joyous. That Sabbath morning, we drove to church with happiness overflowing. Gleefully I signed the church's guest book, "Tom Becraft and his wife-to-be, Bonnie." As our names were read out to the congregation during the welcoming of guests, hearts and hands broke into exuberant celebration with us. Yet, no one could be happier than I, the recipient of love from a winsome, wooing friend! I like it that I was chosen!

God's wooing and choosing is likewise expressed in lover's language. Jesus' parable is about intimately belonging. "Remain in me and I will remain in you" (John 15:4, *HCSB*). "I chose you" (John 15:16, *HCSB*). These words convey a sense of God's intentionality and purpose. He wants us in community with himself in transformative ways.

Abiding in Jesus is not a passive experience. What Jesus is really saying is this: "I've got you, I get you, I grasp you, I sustain you. I am continually with you. Just as I grip you, hang on for My dear life for I will not let you go without blessing you." We thrive and become productive when we grasp God's heart and God's goodness grips us.

Like a tree in its season, we become productive toward our outer world, manifesting love, joy, peace, and other winsome qualities in God's time. Significantly, our maturation occurs not in isolation but in togetherness, and not according to our timetable, but in God's season.

The Vinedresser brings us not only into relationship with himself, but also with others who like ourselves were once down in smelly compost. Through connectedness to Jesus we are linked to one another. In this relationship, love starts from down deep in the earth like sap that sweetens fruit. It ascends out of darkness and through the Christ into an ever-expanding radius of new life bringing a powerful sense of wholeness.

But, not all is easy. Like limbs on a tree we might bump against one another in chaffing, abrasive ways, especially when winds are strong. If we are hit in sensitive places – like where we've been pruned by the Vinedresser – we might decide, "Enough! I'm out of here!" Yet, the Vinedresser knows what we need. I need to shelter and be sheltered by others. When I separate myself from those who have hurt or offended me, I break God's heart and wound God's community.

The Lord's call to remain in relationship with Himself contains a mandate to view others through the centrality of grace. Like branches on a tree, some fellow adherents might be attached to God from a different perspective or angle. This means that the fullness of another person's relationship with God might not be visible from where we are. In fact, the most distant branches, those on the extreme opposite edge, may be seen and known only through the centrality of Christ. As the trunk of his community, Jesus stands between us and those whom we might judge harshly. Or who might judge us.

Strange as it seems, perhaps the most overlooked lesson of Jesus' midnight message is this: Branches on the tree might grow in different directions, but the Director of the direction is not us. Rather, that is the Vinedresser's role. God did not make us the managers of each other's spiritual productivity! Our primary task is to abide in the One who alone is able to bring fruitfulness. The Sacred One provides what is necessary to bring all to Himself, and to give the inheritance of joy to all who rest in Him.

PARTING THE HAIR AND DAD-GUMMING IT

In my travels I've seen combs made out of all kinds of substances, including wood. Some are ornate, some are simple, and all have multiple teeth if they remain true to their purpose. Have you ever tried to part your hair with a one-toothed comb? Isn't it about as effective as combing your hair with a toothpick? The single-toothed comb may be adequate to temporarily scratch an itch, but it's not good for much more!

What would happen if people stayed present to each other, accepting their place in God's hands as grace-aligned instruments of beautification? What would happen to the whirled peas of our babyhood and to the fleas of our adult associations if we allowed God to apply His skill to making us presentable for heaven's royal chambers?

My father-in-law, Norman, was a denture-wearing man when he and Mom came to live with Bonnie and me in Hawaii. Though he was then a hospice patient in a terminal decline, he yet shared his smile with us, sometimes with his dentures in and sometimes without. The difference was remarkable. One evening as he wrapped his smile around some slices of papaya he realized that his teeth were still on his nightstand. He looked up sorrowfully with his chin approaching his nose.

"Dad, gum it!" I said, and Dad laughed and gummed it and gummed it until Mom brought him his teeth. Dad's winsome spirit enlivened my days. His teeth might be missing, but his smile taught me about alignment with what really matters. He cherished each moment, relishing quirkiness even as he prepared his heart for everlasting feasts with God. I miss Dad and celebrate his gracious capacity to "gum it" through the thick and thin of what life offered him.

Gaps in the gums and toothless combs tell stories of brokenness, loss and loneliness. But, does a snaggle-toothed mouth or broken comb tell the whole story? Indeed, whether in a mouth or a comb, teeth are only part of something larger. Likewise we belong to something greater than ourselves. More precisely, we know to whom we belong and that He is more than a broken body. He is altogether lovely, grinning and bearing us all the way home.

BLESSINGS OF THE BROKEN BODY

On the night before his crucifixion, Jesus reclined with his apostles at a low table and said, "I have been *very eager* to eat this Passover meal with you..." (Luke 22:15, *NLT,* emphasis supplied). This sounds to me like a small child's anticipation of Christmas morning. Yet, the context is one of suffering. How can joy and pain converge at such a time?

Jesus proceeds to tell his disciples, "I won't eat this meal again until its meaning is fulfilled in the Kingdom of God." And then He commands, "Eat this meal in order to remember me" (Luke 22:16, *NLT*).

What is Jesus really, *really* talking about? For example, is Jesus alluding to God's message to Isaiah, the prophet? "This is the kind of fasting I want: 'Free those who are wrongly imprisoned; lighten the burden of those who work for you. Let the oppressed go free, and remove the chains that bind people. Share your food with the hungry, and give shelter to the homeless. Give clothes to those who need them, and do not hide from relatives who need your help, then your salvation will come like the dawn and your wounds will quickly heal'" (Isaiah 58:6-8. *NLT*). Is this what Christ's Last Supper's pledge is all about? Will Jesus fast by doing these things?

Or is Jesus reminding of a day spent alongside Lake Galilee eating bread broken and multiplied in his hands? When Jesus fed the 5,000, there is a significant pause in the account. After the miracle, without explanation, Jesus "slipped away into the hills by himself" (John 6:15, *NLT*). Jesus has not announced his kingship as they now think he should. So, the disciples go their own direction, feeling forsaken. In the darkness of that night as a gale sweeps down upon their little boat, Jesus appears to them walking upon tumultuous water. Jesus cries out, "Don't be afraid. I am here!" What a pause! These words are sandwiched between the miracle of the bread's multiplication and the explanation of the bread. They capture the essence of what the bread is all about.

Now the disciples are "eager to let him in the boat" (John 6:21, *NLT*). Immediately they arrive on shore and Jesus unfolds the meaning of the bread. "I am the bread of life...I have come down out of heaven to do the will of God who sent me" and "Anyone who eats this bread will live forever" (John 6:6-53, *NLT*).

Jesus' reference to Himself as bread descended from heaven is a clear allusion to an old familiar story. The Israelites were journeying from Egypt to Canaan, tarrying along the way. They got hungry, and cried out with many complaints for mercy. Grace appeared to them like dew upon dry ground. As the sun crept over the eastern horizon, they peered out from their tents into the rising heat and cried out, "Manna!" meaning, "What is it?" What they saw was a mysterious resource for living. Gathered into containers, it could be seasoned, baked, boiled, and savored as heavenly food.

This life-saving food became representative of a collaborative relationship between the Israelites and the Source of Life. So significant was it to the existence and salvation of the Israelite people that a pot of manna was housed at the heart of the Tabernacle, within the Ark of the Covenant, *at the precise center* of the Hebrew encampment. The manna was *always* central to their communion with God and with one another.

The manna shared a place within the Covenant Box alongside the Ten Commandments and Aaron's almond staff that had inexplicably bloomed back to life after dying. The manna in the pot spoke of heavenly mercies that could be received or rejected. Collectively, the rod, manna and commandments show how God saves.

Significantly, these three items came to the Israelites in a particular order. First, came Aaron's staff representing God's choice to raise the dead. Then came the manna, an expression of His soul-empowerment; and finally came the Ten Commandments. This order is meaningful for a number of reasons, particularly as we examine how God invites people to accept the outpouring of his favor. God's grace calls, *then* imparts strength, and *then* draws toward faith-filled obedience.

In this journey of transformation, it is no small gift that the provision of manna is linked to a Sabbath rest *even before* the Sabbath Commandment was placed in the Decalogue on tablets of stone. (After all, Sabbath was the climactic appointment of creation week, *before* sin entered, and long before Abraham, Isaac, Jacob and Moses were even born.) God said, "In the morning you will have all the bread you want. Then you will know that I am the Lord your God" (Exodus 16:11, *NLT*).

Through this mysterious gift, God provided affirmation of His nearness to them. The nomads stepped outside their tents and saw food for which they had not labored. There had been no plowing, no sowing of seed, no fertilizing, and no weeding. It was all undeserved and abundant! All they needed to do was stretch out hands to receive what God placed before them. *Through the giving of grace in this manner, God declared that He holds space for all humankind to rest and to be restored.*

What did God ask of them? Only that they live and harvest in a way that acknowledged and accepted His grace! The posture of harvesting is on one's knees. The attitude is gratitude.

The provision of the bread is the story of God's ongoing creation and sustaining grace. This is evident in God's instructions about when and how to gather the manna. Make first things first, gathering grace at daybreak. Attend to yourself, your family and your neighbors by taking only what is needed. Don't hoard because greed corrupts and stinks. Most of all, attend to the Creator. As you heed the Creator, the Creator will supply all your needs – including rest!

At the heart of God's instructions regarding the gathering of the manna was a call to honor God by honoring his Sabbath gift. "This is what the Lord commanded, 'Tomorrow will be a day of complete rest, a holy Sabbath day set apart for the Lord. So bake or boil *as much as you want* today and set it apart for tomorrow'" (Exodus 16:23, *NLT,* emphasis supplied).

The weekly Sabbath could not approach unnoticed for manna marked the time. On the sixth day of each week, God granted a super sufficiency of bread upon the ground. God gave a double blessing on the Preparation Day, turning the hearts of his people toward a bounteous rest the next day. If there were doubts in any minds about what day God hallowed, it became clear to them through tangible, observable blessings. He made His presence unquestionably clear to them every sixth day as His Sabbath approached. The Sabbath was preceded each week by a Day of Promise, the sixth day. It was to be a time of anticipatory joy.

On any other day of the week, gathering manna beyond one's needs resulted in maggot-infestations and a horrifying stench. But, on the sixth day, God commanded each person to collect *according to the heart's desire.* This collecting did not result in any kind of rot. As the community awakened on Sabbath morning the preserved purity of the bread testified to an important truth from God: "Don't be afraid. I am here." What a way to end and start a new week. Through His Sabbath gift, God holds time and space every week for everyone to claim a new life.

Wind back the clock now. On Thursday night (corresponding to the Biblical start of God's Day of Promise) we gather around Jesus in the Upper Room. We watch Jesus take the bread and break it. In His face we see ancient and recent history come into the present to say, Sabbath rest is here. We see God providing sustenance morning after morning in the desert. We see the 5,000 whom Jesus fed. In these moments, as we look at Jesus, we know the fullness of the manna. The "what is it" mystery of the manna is embodied in the personhood of the Broken Bread, the Body of Christ.

Indeed, the Apostle John saw and heard Jesus in vision, saying 70 years *after* his ascension: "To everyone who is victorious I will give some of the manna that has been hidden away in heaven" (Revelation 2:17, *NLT*). There is manna, past and present. Long ago the people of God were fed by bread that that was was preserved unto and throughout the Sabbath. Today, in the same way we are saved by a Savior who does not grow stale. He is the Living Bread for all eternity. He comes with healing power. He comes to bring justice, mercy, and rest. He comes from His heavenly sanctuary to make His love for us concrete.

Along with the heavenly bread, Jesus promises, "I will give to each one a white stone and on the white stone will be engraved a new name that no one understands except the one who receives it" (Revelation 2:17, *NLT*). As one who has occasionally grappled with depression, this evokes hope within me for several reasons.

First, in the Greco-Roman culture of John's time, a small white pebble carried the weight of a giant boulder in determining the outcome of one's life. When called to stand before a Roman judge, one's fate was dropped into the hand in the form of an impermeable rock. A black stone proclaimed guilt and called for death's darkness. A white stone proclaimed innocence and assured ascent from a dungeon into glorious light and life.

In the Book of Revelation God's people stand robed in white garments as they come before God's Mercy Seat. The whiteness of God's courtroom is no dull, flat, non-reflective white, but is the scintillating, glistening, magnificent hue of heaven. Let there be no dark doubts about the color of forgiveness! The white stone dispels all uncertainties about our salvation.

Second, throughout the ancient world, it was common for persons to carry a stone as a talisman or charm to ward off evil. It was believed that one might gain power or control over a deity by etching that god's name upon the stone and keeping it upon one's person. Furthermore, the amulet's power was doubled if only its owner knew that name. By carrying the good-luck stone, one could walk each day in freedom.

At least, that is what people thought. Jesus says to John, there is a name that transcends the superstitions of magical thinking, and I give that name to ALL who receive the holy bread. Jesus promises that there is no restricting of the power of His name to just a few. In essence He says, "Let all who fearfully carry a secret talisman for good luck know that they are safe in life and in death, not because of the amulet, but because God makes Himself known through Jesus, the Christ."

Finally, the white stone declares that heaven belongs to those who prevail when battered and bruised and broken in life's arena. In the Greco-Roman culture, slaves were sometimes cast before lions, or thrust into unwanted battles in the coliseum to test their endurance. Those who conquered were rewarded with a small white stone, a *tessera*, upon which were written the letters SP, which "stands for the Latin word *spectatus* which means *a man whose courage has been proved beyond a doubt*" (William Barclay, *The Revelation of John*, Volume 1, p. 96). Christ's white stone is a passport to citizenship and privilege as a free person in a new world. I want that new world!

The newness in the new earth is about much more than a point in time; it is especially about quality. In Jesus I encounter the substance of superlative grace and am energized to know that heaven's gifts are accessible and perfectly fresh for my daily needs. As I struggle with the realities of everyday life in a fractured world, my heart cries out that God will bring strength and healing to *all* his people, including me. I want that ancient newness NOW!

In these moments of yearning, I hear the Apostle Paul proclaim, "God raised us up from the dead along with Christ Jesus and seated us with him in the heavenly realms because we are united with Christ" (Ephesians 2:6. *NLT*). What a paradoxical statement! My feet are stuck on *terra firma*, but I'm *already* in heaven. How can it be that I am part of an earthly community that transcends this earth! The answer is found "in the incredible wealth of God's grace and kindness toward us, as shown to us in all he has done for us who are united with Jesus Christ" (Ephesians 2:7, *NIV*).

FINDING NEWNESS EACH DAY

Recently a veteran nurse stopped me in the corridor of the Intensive Care Unit and asked me to check in with a new nurse. "Her patient died last night and this was her first death," she said. She then added, "We never forget our first."

So, I went looking for Tillie. No matter the circumstances, death causes an emotional response. Tillie's tears trickled down. I was aware that the death of virtual strangers often impacts profoundly, causing an examination of life's meaning and purpose. Why do we care when someone dies? Is it simply that the death of another person triggers feelings of our own mortality? Or is it because that person never really lived? Or is it because we're torn by mysteries of the vast unknown?

Indeed, I have not forgotten the first human corpse that I saw. Far from home, I was walking on a beach in Pusan, South Korea, when I noticed a cluster of somber and agitated people at the water's edge. Drawing closer I saw what they saw: a middle-aged man who had washed up on the sand after several days in the water. Bloated and putrefied, he was not a pretty sight. In that instant of shock, I felt a visceral awareness that death is an ugly enemy.

Yet in those moments I experienced an inward stirring of hope. The Apostle Paul declares, "These dying bodies cannot inherit what will last forever. But let me reveal to you a wonderful secret. We will not all die, but we will be transformed...Our dying bodies must be transformed into bodies that will never die...Christ must reign...and the last enemy to be destroyed is death...When our dying bodies have been transformed into bodies that will never die, this Scripture will be fulfilled: 'Death is swallowed up in victory'" (1 Corinthians 15:26, 53, *NLT*).

Just as every human body is a community of cells, capable of mysterious and marvelous functioning or disintegration, every person is part of something larger than self and has the potentiality of life or death. The breakdown of wellbeing is countered by an infinite infusion of divine mercy. "God is so rich in mercy, and he loved us so much, that even though we were dead in our sins, he gave us life when he raised Christ from the dead...We are God's masterpiece. He has created us anew in Christ Jesus, so we can do the good things he planned long ago" (Ephesians 2:4, 8, *NLT*).

What does this mystery of newness mean? Paul explains, "Christ himself brought peace to us...He made peace between Jews and Gentiles by creating in himself one new people...Together as one body, Christ reconciled both groups to God..." (Ephesians 2:14-16, *NLT*).

Newness is about how we live in community. Here is the essence of this community: "We will speak the truth in love, growing in every way more and more like Christ, who is the head of his body, the church. He makes the whole body fit together perfectly. As each part does its special work, it helps the other part grow, so that the whole body is healthy and growing and full of love" (Ephesians 4:15,16, *NLT*).

There are times when I am sorely disturbed by the dysfunctions that I see in the world around me, both among believers and those who make no profession of faith. Can authentic love be found anywhere? I want to scream, Why? Though I love people, sometimes I don't "like" them. In those moments, I am called back to myself. Who am I to judge? My own failures are real to me, and sometimes I don't like myself. Thankfully, enfeebled and defective as we are, we are never apart from a God who cares.

It was the Sunday before Christmas when I received a letter that turned my world upside down. The wounding of my spirit was so profound that I doubted that I would ever heal. I felt ravaged by feelings of betrayal, bitterness, anger, and self-disgust. I felt unloved, and unlovable. Yet, life must go on!

Sabbath came and I had to preach a Holy Communion message. My sermon preparation was a reflection of my inner void. Both it and I felt inadequate. As I sat behind the communion altar with the sacred emblems spread out before me, I wrestled with my inner turmoil. How could I speak anything out of my desolated spirit? What could I possibly say that would be of value to anyone?

Congregants sang a hymn as they gathered following our traditional foot-washing service. The table was spread before me; platters of freshly baked unleavened bread at my left hand and unfermented grape juice at my right awaited distribution to my church family. Feelings of unworthiness tugged at my heart as the hymn ended.

Yet, in those moments I heard words coming unbidden from my mouth into the microphone: "On the table before us today we have a message from the heart of God. The bread and the fruit of the grape that we are about to receive are emblems of God's great love toward us. They represent the arms of God reaching out to us with the hug of heaven. They are God's arms saying, 'I love you.' So, receive the bread and the wine now as God's loving and forgiving embrace."

Moments later, as elders distributed the emblems, I saw Erin, a three-year old toddler, squirm out of her mother's arms in the rear pew and move down the center aisle toward the front. Arms reached out to capture her, but she eluded them all. Her eyes fastened on me as she pumped her little legs with increasing intensity. No football player in a championship game could have covered the distance with more drive. She reached the communion altar, climbed over the lap of an elder sitting beside me, and threw her arms in the air in celebration before wrapping them around my neck in a tight embrace. She hugged me and hugged me some more as she repeatedly whispered into my ear, "Pastor Tom, I love you, and so does God." She and her message nestled into my heart calling me back from the dead. Thank God for such relentless grace!

Crossing the Ice as a Leader

I felt and heard the sound in the same instant. Ice cracked beneath my five-year old feet. From the shore my older brother Jim screamed, "Run!" Frantically, I scrabbled and scrambled for footing as water seeped upward from the winter pond soaking my boots. Fear burst from my mouth in vaporous puffs of panic. I was not where I was supposed to be.

Mom had warned us. "Do NOT go near the pond." But, Jim was an experienced veteran of mother's worries. He navigated in and around her cautions with the aplomb of a little general. "Come on," he had told me. "She'll never know."

He was a leader. I was just a follower. He had crossed over the ice first, and then urged me to follow, asserting that it was "really thick." And it nearly cost me my life. Not that Jim was/is a bad guy. It's simply that neither of us then discerned what leadership is all about. Where ice is thin and waters are deep beneath it takes more than bravado and bold assertiveness to secure the far shore.

Jim and I lived to learn about the role of grace in leadership. While grace is often described as "unmerited mercy and undeserved kindness," it also has an instructive element that transforms choices.

Notice how Scripture describes grace: "For the grace of God has appeared that offers salvation to all people. It teaches us to say 'No' to ungodliness and worldly passions, and to live self-controlled, upright and godly lives in this present age while we wait for the blessed hope – the appearing of the glory of our great God and Savior, Jesus Christ" (Titus 2:11-13 NCV).

Grace is herein personified as a rabbi, a sensei, our teacher and guide, instructing us to put boundaries in place against that which is harmful or unjust or destructive of self and others. It calls us to discern what is holy and to model justice and mercy. It anticipates ultimate goodness in the appearance of God to all and for all.

Grace's inclusivity summons caregivers to care wisely. Occasionally this means advocacy for the voiceless. We give voice to others when we speak for justice. We give voice when we provide space and opportunity for their voices to be heard. We give voice when we join our voices with those whose whisper is barely heard. We give voice by listening deeply to the undercurrents of people's lives and provide channels for their dreams to flow and bubble to the surface of life.

Sometimes grace means harnessing the energy of anger. Neville was dying on the Intensive Care Unit. Grieving family members surrounded him. They had fought alongside him for weeks, hoping that his decline could be reversed. All systems were shutting down. Kidneys, lungs, heart, liver, and mind. Neville could not speak for himself. So, his family spoke for him, stating that he would not want to be kept alive on machines any longer with no hope of regaining his former vitality. Therefore, the care team reverently removed the breathing tube, titrating medication to keep his breathing comfortable without hastening death. His spirit/breath moved in and out slowly saying good-bye to family.

It was during this sacred vigil that a physician blustered into the patient's room. "You must stop this," he said. "What you are doing is inhumane. There are still things we can do."

The family reacted with horror and anger. My own instantaneous anger at the doctor's verbal insensitivity compelled me to immediately exert myself in ways that are at odds with my usual non-confrontational demeanor. When the disruptive doctor pivoted on his heels and left to talk to the physician in charge of the unit, I took the family to an adjacent room where I listened to their anguish. I then waded into conversations with a hospital administrator, members of the immediate care team, and the vigil-breaking doctor.

From an ethical standpoint, the issue was not about legalities and liabilities, or about what doctors, chaplains, nurses, or family members wanted, but about how Neville might move toward wholeness in the face of his terminal condition. Conversations were animated and patient-focused.

Scripture teaches that authentic grace says "No" to what is wrong, and "Yes" to what is right. Thus, protection of others from abuse becomes a dimension of grace. So, we seek compassion at every turn, confronting wrongs by speaking truth in love. Such caring is not blind. It assesses needs and responds from a place of open-eyed awareness toward what heals and what destroys. Such grace is rooted in knowledge of one's own limitations.

The next morning as I was about to start my shift, I heard a knock on my office door. The previous night's vigil-breaker stood before me with eyes and face projecting an absence of sleep. Regret was palpable both in his demeanor and in his words. He apologized. I saw him in those moments as a wounded healer, capable now of leading more compassionately toward ultimate wellness. Looking in the doc's face, I realized we'd crossed an important threshold together. We faced each other with compassion, respect and commitment, leaders who know the agonies and joys of leadership.

Leadership at the Most Elemental Level

Authentic leadership is not defined by job title, high position within the strata of an organizational flow chart, or by public acclaim. Rather, real leadership happens at the most elemental level. It happens when we become self-reflective and create room for others to grasp possibilities. It happens when we seek inner growth for ourselves, and when we allow for the growth of others. It happens when we hold ourselves accountable, and when we give others latitude to pursue their own pathway toward wholeness.

Real leadership for transformation can be modeled by persons in prominent positions, but it may also be seen among those who work outside the glare of spotlights. I've watched persons, regardless of job description, contribute to the reshaping of caregiving, making their surroundings more patient-centered. Whether prominent or unknown, true leaders hold space for people around them to achieve their full potential as children of the Sacred. They become committed to showing respect both toward themselves and toward others as recipients of the Divine's life blood. This quality of leadership is not determined by position or title.

Tim, my younger brother, is a scholar who has studied the dynamics of transformative leadership. With his permission, here is an essay he wrote and shared with me recently:

Words are versatile, full of diverse reference and inviting ambiguity. Such reference and ambiguity, however, are often masked by common usage. The nouns "leader" and "leadership", for example, often conjure images of hierarchical and dependent relationships. Our leaders are presidents and senators, CEOs and the titled nobility of our generation. Their successes are our adulation; their failures are our suffering. Our leaders account for our progress or our malaise—our condition pivots on the lives they lead.

Such images are often further bathed in notions of birthright and situation. Leaders are born to fulfill destiny. Leaders are created by situation and circumstance. Leaders lead unique lives and travel through unique terrain. The lives they lead touch those who follow, but their lives are substantively different. The terrain they travel may also cradle others, but they walk and rock to a different lullaby. They are a breed apart. They are men and women uniquely called. They are the lucky few.

While these images accurately reflect a type of leader and leadership, they in no way exhaust the inherent referential possibilities. The underlying verb, "to lead", suggests that those aspiring to lead others need not depend on hierarchical relationships encouraging dependency. To lead, after all, is to show the way to a destination by going in advance. This means that he or she who leads may do so by compelling example rather than by compelling position. He or she who leads others may do so by leading a worthy life, a life worth emulating.

This underlying verb further suggests that leadership is the birthright of all, regardless of situation. To lead a life, after all, is to live a life - but to lead a life is far more suggestive than to simply live one. To lead a life suggests that one willfully guides and directs his or her own behavior and experience rather than being mindlessly dependent on others for guidance and direction. To lead a life suggests a person proactive within situation and circumstance rather than a person buffeted helplessly by either. To lead a life proactively suggests a life worth living, a life worth emulating.

Such leadership, while the birthright of all, is perhaps a road less traveled. The terrain through which we all travel often encourages dependency and abdication of personal responsibility. The inner terrain within which we all live is closer than a heartbeat and is hard to see. Enticed by the first, by thoroughfares of received wisdom and highways of little resistance, we careen helter-skelter toward destinations unchosen and often unknown, without map or compass, ignoring the second.

If each of us is to accept our birthright as leaders we must step beyond first-take understandings of outer terrain - beyond unanalyzed acceptance of its thoroughfares and highways - towards greater cartographic responsibility. We must map the terrain through which we pass, and which we certainly influence, if we are to arrive at any self-chosen destination. We must further recognize that this terrain changes daily, and that we must therefore not make our understandings inviolable.

If we are to accept our birthright as leaders we must also step beyond ignorance of inner terrain - beyond the dulling cacophony and blurring proximity of inner being - towards a cartography of self. We must map our inner being if we are to understand that which animates and motivates our lives, if we are to understand our own behavior. We must map inner being if we are to lead lives with eyes open to inner light and shadow, if we are to step beyond self-absorbed and dependent living, if we are to step into the true light of being. We must map our inner being if we are to legitimately lead others by example through the vagaries of outer terrain - terrain changing, in the Buddhist phrase, as rapidly as the flames of a house on fire - towards a destination chosen by all.

We must also remember that self-cartography is never over. Self-mastery is ephemeral, a moving target. If we are to lead, if we are to accept our birthright, we must not simply be once born or twice born, but rather, must be reborn daily. We must continuously transcend not only our self-understandings, but we must also continuously transcend, or transform, that which we are. This is the core challenge facing those who would lead and teach others, the challenge of helping others by going in advance, the challenge of leading a life worth living. (Tim Becraft, ©2012, used by permission).

A Life Worth Honoring

I awakened in the dark this morning, September 22, with tears in my eyes. Daddy is dying. Last night I carried him to bed, changed his diapers, dressed him in warm pajamas, and then tucked him in for the night. His thin arms wrapped weakly around my neck as I lifted him. As I laid him down, his stubbly cheek rubbed against my own, rubbing raw my emotions. I miss my Father, the man who leaped high fences and climbed tall mountains, that gentle soul whose heart has loved so deeply. Today, I'm not a chaplain. I'm a son and a brother, swimming with my brothers and sisters in a sea of grief. The currents are strong, and I feel the pull of an undertow.

Last night while my siblings and I encircled his bed, our mother nestled alongside Daddy, no longer remembering his name, but knowing that he is "that special guy." Her confused mind reached out hands to touch and caress his face. Their sixty-five years of togetherness has shaped a family that loves them. We simultaneously want them to experience release from bodily aches and pains, but do not want to lose them.

Since Mom and Dad came to live with my sister two years ago, Sue has tucked them in bed every night with a ritual, singing a song learned in our childhood. Last night we sang together, "Tis love that makes us happy...Tis love that smooths the way...Tis love that keeps us kind to others every day." As my mouth struggled to find the words, I thought, love is not always smooth. But, it does make pain more bearable.

I ponder the nature of caregiving. Caregiving is exhausting under even the best of circumstances. As Mom and Dad's primary caregivers, my sister Sue and Lee, my brother-in-law, are especially weary. They have attended to Mom and Dad day and night with unwavering gentleness for two years now. They care deeply and passionately. The threat of burnout is very real. Yet, I know that they and the rest of my family will not stop caring. Why? Because our parents have given us anchor points to which we return as a caring unit when we are stretched to the limits of our endurance.

We are convicted that faith, hope and love transcend death. The heaviness of grief and loss is real to each of us. But, we live with anticipation of a life beyond pain, suffering and burnout. Our love is rooted and grounded in a faith that was implanted in our hearts through countless stories of the Sacred Presence and a "blessed hope." As God was real to Mom and Dad, God is real to us in these moments.

~~~~~~~

Three days later I am once again awakened in the dark. It is September 25. There is a gentle tapping on my door. Sue stands in front of me, tears streaming down her face as she quietly sobs, "He's gone."

In a few days there will be a funeral. So, we children gather to make plans. Years ago my parents picked out songs and scriptures and asked me to officiate. But today I do not want to be a clergy person. I just want to simply be a son and a brother. As we swap stories, my younger brother Tim tells of an interview he did of Dad for a graduate school class 20 years ago. It was about leadership and change. Collectively, we determine that nothing would honor Dad more than to listen to and heed his voice responding to questions from one of his sons. Here is Tim at the memorial service:

Conversing about Servant Leadership

All of us have memories of those still with us and of those who have left us. We often nurture and massage those memories, and even construct language formalizing their content and meaning. Such memories often sustain us, guide us, and help us choose how we wish to live. They often lead us, influencing how we lead our lives. My memories of my father are such memories. Some help me smile, some help me laugh, some profoundly move me, and nearly all help me choose how I hope to lead my own life, even though I frequently fall short.

Later today many of you will share your own memories of him, and we will smile, laugh, cry, and be profoundly moved. Some of you may tell of Bob plunging from great heights on hot days into deep and cooling waters, filled with childlike joy, or of him jumping barbed wire fences while still in slacks, to our mother's considerable agitation, or of him seated backwards on the handlebars of a bicycle and peddling down a gravel driveway, to the delight and wonder of the children watching, or of him growing a mustache after falling from those handlebars and injuring his upper lip, or of him riding again, with a stiff upper lip.

And I could tell you of how moved I was hearing him read, only several months ago, in a weak but sure voice, "Yea, though I walk through the valley of the shadow of death, I will fear no evil: For thou art with me; Thy rod and thy staff they comfort me. Thou preparest a table before me in the presence of mine enemies: Thou anointest my head with oil; my cup runneth over; Surely goodness and mercy shall follow me all the days of my life: And I will dwell in the house of the LORD forever" (Psalm 23, KJV).

I could also tell of being deeply moved when I witnessed Lee supporting Dad on his arm, when Dad could hardly ambulate, in the way Dad supported both his parents, or of being deeply moved seeing Tom carrying Dad in his arms on Dad's last day, in the way Dad carried us when we were children.

What some of us may struggle to find is the stories he told or the things he said, because he was a man of few words, even though he loved language and was articulate and wise when he chose to speak. What I really want to share is Dad's own voice, a voice often unheard, by sharing his answers to questions I asked him nearly two decades ago.

My siblings, can you help me? Tom, can you provide Daddy's voice as I ask the questions Dad answered so long ago? Jim, can you be the historian when needed?

LEADERSHIP INFLUENCES

Tim: *Who has most influenced your understanding of leadership?*

Dad: *My father and my grandfather.*

Tim: *How did your father influence you?*

Dad: *He always had strong feelings for the unfortunate. He was honest and loyal. He would take time for people, time to talk, time to listen. He was sensitive to feelings. We were his first concern. Sometimes he pushed us children though. Pushing is not leading. He tried to harmonize his public and private life. He showed steadiness, fairness, and liberalism.*

Jim: *Virgil Becraft, Dad's father was a pastor, college Bible teacher, and hospital chaplain in California and the Pacific Northwest.*

Tim: *What about Grandpa Burg?*

Dad: *He was honest. He had feelings for the needs of others, seen often in his commitment to teaching and to people. His goodness!*

Jim: *Like his son-in-law Virgil, Francis Burg, was also a longtime minister and college professor.*

Tim: *What events have influenced your understanding of leadership?*

Dad: *I don't know. Leadership is not an event. Leadership is people.*

Jim: *Notice! Dad used the plural – people!*

Tim: *What formal leadership roles have you had?*

Dad: *I've been a church deacon and elder...I didn't always feel comfortable in those roles...Real leadership is taking responsibilities not assigned, carrying responsibilities without being asked.*

Tim: *What informal leadership roles have you had?*

Dad: I suppose my family.

Jim: In the original interview, at this point, Mom interjected, commenting on Dad's stabilizing influence within the church, his steadiness, his values, his morals, his steadfast vision, his influence within the immediate and extended family.

Tim: What are your current formal leadership roles?

Dad: I'm retired!

Tim: What are your current informal leadership roles?

Dad: Helping those in the community who need help; being a parent.

LEADERSHIP AND SELF CONCEPT

Tim: How do you see yourself as a leader?

Dad: I'm willing to do my best even if my capacity is limited. I'm willing to accept support – I have a good support system. I'm persistent. I'm not a quitter. I don't want to take on too much at once. I want to complete something first. I want to participate rather than just watch. I want to be involved.

Tim: What are your weaknesses as a leader?

Dad: I am not aggressive enough, but aggressiveness is a two-edged sword. Self-confidence – my history persists! But, I've made progress toward self-acceptance...self-esteem. Initiative to follow through on an idea. For example, the silver business was full of opportunity, but I was conservative.

Jim: When we were young, Daddy collected old x-ray film and the solutions in which the film was processed. He sold the film to a refiner and extracted silver from the solutions by machines he purchased. He recovered many hundreds of pounds of silver over the years. As he approached retirement, his boss, Dr. Martin, expressed concern about the silver and our family's safety. Dad reassured him, saying, "It's all in a safe place." At that time he had just one coffee can full of silver under the kitchen sink. The rest he had sold to pay for our education. In other words, we kids were "a *safe place." Dad measured wealth by what he was able to impart to the hearts and minds of his children.*

Tim: *How do you address your weaknesses?*

Dad: *I have developed more relaxed relationships. This has been gradual, not a particular effort. This change has come from a spouse who has confidence in me, and from my children. To change we must have a need to change, a desire to change, a willingness to change.*

LEADERSHIP DEFINITIONS

Tim: *What is your definition of a leader?*

Dad: *Someone who doesn't try to do everything himself but who enlists the help of others toward a common goal, someone who doesn't want to credit self but who wants others to feel they have achieved, someone who allows others to contribute. A leader doesn't need blind followers!*

Tim: *What is your definition of a follower?*

Dad: *A positive follower is someone who recognizes the attributes of a good leader and who is supportive of that leader. A negative follower is totally dependent on the other.*

Tim: *How are leaders and followers different?*

Dad: *They, to a certain extent, must have the same qualities – honesty, fair play, loyalty, not being lazy, cooperating with each other, giving of themselves, giving credit to each other. They are supportive of each other – they are interdependent. They are considerate of each other's needs.*

LEADERSHIP OF SELF

Tim: *How does leading one's own life relate to leading other people?*

Dad: *One must be true to self. One must choose whom to follow. If one chooses to lead, one must choose virtues rather than otherwise, integrity rather than subversive thoughts or behavior. If one follows, one must choose a leader who allows choices, initiative, and suggestions.*

LEADERSHIP OF OTHERS

Tim: *How does self-understanding relate to leading others?*

Dad: *If you understand your own strengths and weaknesses, if you know where you want to go, and how you want to get there, you can have faith in direction, you can have the compassion necessary for relating to others – empathy starts with self-understanding.*

Dad never aspired to leadership, but he led a good life, and in so doing led us and influenced us and enriched us in countless ways. He climbed to great heights and plunged into cool waters with childlike joy, but never risked family or friends. He sometimes fell, but always rode again. He has led many beside still waters; he has led in the paths of righteousness. Though Dad is now absent, he is present within us. He led, and still leads those who remember. (Interview ©2012, by Tim Becraft; used by permission).

It has been said that the difference between an estate and a legacy is the difference between what is in one's bank account and what endures in the hearts of those we love after we die.

Dad's legacy? Immeasurable!

Chapter 3

LEARNING LIFE'S LESSONS

INTEGRATING THE DIVINE AND HUMAN

An overhead announcement summoned me to the emergency department where a trauma team was tending to a young woman who had just shot herself in the head while playing Russian roulette with a friend. Her handgun sent a bullet into her brain causing a massive non-survivable injury. Brain scans showed a flat line, indicating that she was now legally dead and therefore a candidate for donating organs to anonymous recipients. A ventilator breathed for her and powerful drugs sustained her heart and blood flow as I escorted her parents upstairs to our Intensive Care Unit where the young woman's body and her grieving family would await the arrival of a transplant team.

In the midst of this vigil, a pink-smocked volunteer knocked lightly on the door and gestured that she needed to speak with me. She showed me a note with two names on it, and said, "There are two ladies out in the lobby who want to come and pray with the patient and the family. What should I tell them?"

I turned to the mother and father, showed them the volunteer's note, and asked for their wishes. Neither parent could identify the two visitors. "Please tell them," the dad said, "that we are grateful for their prayers. But, now is not a good time here and we are limiting visitors just to family." He further voiced a fear that other family members might learn of the tragedy from strangers before he and the mom could contact them. They asked me to find out who the two visitors were and how they had learned of the patient's accident.

With this mandate, I entered the lobby and was instantly greeted by two women whose faces were full of concern. "How is she? Can we see her? We heard it's bad." They hardly paused to hear me as they tried to navigate around me down the corridor toward the death vigil.

I held my ground, and they evaded answering my own questions.

"Please sit back down. I need you to remain here," I said.

"But, can you tell us," they asked. "Did you lead her in the sinner's prayer? You need to do that before it's too late. And, we've already launched several prayer chains. We've got a bunch of people praying for her. We've got her on several prayer chains now..."

Uh-oh!

Bound by confidentiality, I responded, "The parents want to thank you for your prayers. But, they ask that you give them this time alone with their daughter. [long pause]. And they ask that you say absolutely nothing to anyone since they have not yet had an opportunity to talk to other family members. I need you to respect the family's privacy."

"But, what about the sinner's prayer?" they asked. "Did she confess her sins and her need for Christ? Did she receive Jesus into her heart as her personal Savior? And what about you? Are you a Christian? Have you been born again? Can you guide her in the sinner's prayer?" I think, *Do they really want answers?*

Before I could speak again, the older of the two women spontaneously bowed her head and burst into a fervent prayer that God would compel me to do the "right thing" and lead the young woman to Christ "before it is too late."

As she ended her petition, I likewise burst into prayer: "Lord, please guide these two ladies safely home and hear their prayers from there. Amen."

They then left.

SEEKING THE HOLY PURPOSE

Nearly every week someone phones or drops by my office to inquire how they might become a chaplain and "do what you do." I have encountered a wide range of perceptions regarding the work of chaplains. Like the two women just mentioned whose agenda clashed with the immediate needs of my patient and her family, some visitors are naïve and clueless regarding what is required to be an effective spiritual caregiver. Others are keenly aware of both human and sacred dynamics. When visitors inquire regarding how one becomes a chaplain, I invite them to consider three elements of God's equipping:

1. **Calling** - Do you believe that God is calling you to this ministry? If so, how is that calling coming to you?
2. **Skill-set** - What equips you for this ministry? In other words, how well do your innate abilities and acquired skills shape your interactions with people when they are experiencing challenges?
3. **Passions** - What energizes you with joy and hope in the face of human pain and suffering? Specifically, who and what holds you as you enter into the chaotic stories of people's lives?

Out of my own experience, I can say that my understanding of God's calling has shifted through the years, and that it has now merged with my passions and skill-set in ways that are life affirming. My sense of calling has deepened, my skills have been honed, and my life has been energized by encounters that affirm God's willingness to enter into the details of my life.

Thus, in this chapter, I want to sketch a picture of how a person's calling, skill-set and passions may converge to equip him or her for ministry. In doing so, I will present snippets of my own journey. But, the story is larger than self. It is ultimately about the Sacred Other. It is about the Holy One who calls, equips, and ultimately energizes with joyful abandon.

Long ago my mother held me on her lap and told me that my life had been spared from an early death for a holy purpose. The tarnished penny in her hand spoke loudly to me of how I nearly died. I had inhaled that coin while pretending to be a vacuum cleaner on the kitchen floor. After surgeons extracted the coin through an incision in my ten-month-old neck, my parents took steps to shelter me from further harm by removing the ingestible button-eyes of my favorite stuffed friends. My teddy bear and his cohorts became sightless. This did not thwart my imagination. Often they were my audience as I exercised my vocal cords in imitation of my preacher grandfather. Their non-responsiveness did not keep me from believing that somehow, in some fashion, I was born to change the world! It was the beginning of my quest for the Holy Purpose.

Audiences have come and gone many times since then. My childish naïveté has likewise slipped into the past. Since then, more than once, I've lain in bed at night pondering the trajectory of my life, both past and future. I've crisscrossed oceans in response to a deeply imbedded sense that God made me a minister, wooing my heart to love and serve Him since I was yet a babe in my mother's arms.

More often than not, I've found satisfaction in my searching. Yet, there have been seasons of upheaval. It sometimes seemed that God placed me where my capabilities and passions were out of sync with what God was requiring of me. It was sometimes painful. So, my perspective today is more seasoned than it was 40 years ago as I was starting life as a minister.

Yet, much can be said about the role of naiveté and innocence. In fact, I believe God uses childlike simplicity to bring us into places where our personhood is molded in ways that are necessary for future usefulness.

Forty years ago, straight out of college, when I received an invitation to pastor a congregation of American military personnel in Okinawa, I instantly and unquestioningly said "Yes" to this assignment even though I had an inner inkling that the "plan" would be changed to something else before I landed on the island.

Sure enough! En route to Naha, the prefectural capitol of Okinawa, I stopped in Tokyo where Japanese church leaders told me that I would spend at least one year, perhaps two, studying Japanese. Six months into this brutal experience, they came to me and said, "We've been thinking, would you be willing to pastor in a Japanese-language church instead of an English-speaking congregation?"

I asked, "Why would you want a *gaijin*, a foreigner, to pastor a Japanese church when you already have over a hundred Japanese pastors?"

They responded, "This is a face-saving culture, and our ministers often hesitate to try something new or different because they don't want to fail publically." They paused and looked at me, seeking my understanding. "But, you are an American, so it won't bother you," they said. "We need someone willing to try different approaches in ministry to show us what might work, even if you might fail along the way."

Thus, in my mind, I came to personify a certain Biblical description: "He chose the fools of the world to confound the wise." For many years, I became the clown outside the Big Top exhorting passersby to enter into the Lord's joy.

Over time, I eventually became an academically trained, field-based cross-culturalist who worked hard as a local church pastor in Japan. My efforts resulted in ever-expanding responsibilities – a national leadership role, then an assignment as an associate professor of applied theology at Japan Saniku Gakuin College. I felt honored and trusted by the people I lived among.

Meanwhile my sons grew up, and family matters eventually required that I say good-bye to Japan and many friends. I returned to America with my family, becoming further immersed in multi-cultural pastorates and educational ministries, first in Seattle, Washington, then in Hawaii. Each time I was reassigned I experienced culture shock and separation from important relationships, both personal and professional. These moves caused waves of grief and loss. It often felt as if a bulldozer had channeled a hole through my heart.

Then came one more bump to my equilibrium.

CLINICAL PASTORAL EDUCATION
AND WHOLENESS

One day I was suddenly unemployed in answer to a heartfelt prayer. Together with my wife, Bonnie Oneonta-Becraft, I had prayed that God would open a way for us to relocate from Hawaii to be closer to our families on the mainland. After 25 years overseas in Korea, Japan, and Hawaii, this prayer was answered when Bonnie was invited to become Director of Pastoral Care at Walla Walla General Hospital in Eastern Washington. I resigned my school chaplaincy and teaching position in Hawaii and accompanied her.

No pastoral or teaching positions were immediately available for me in our new location. Thus, in the dark of the night, without my accustomed roles and responsibilities, I wondered: Who am I?

I sensed that my personal identity had become wrapped up in roles and responsibilities. I needed to find and reclaim my core self. Bonnie wisely suggested that I utilize my "sabbatical" to pursue professional and personal growth by enrolling in a Clinical Pastoral Education (CPE) course for chaplains, a process that became both life-affirming and life-directing.

So, what is CPE? It is:
- An action-reflection process of education in which a group of peers covenant to attend to one's own and each other's giftedness and brokenness in a quest for personal and professional wellness as spiritual caregivers (See the Association of Clinical Pastoral Education's website: http://www.acpe. edu/).
- A process of personal theological integration and grounding, equipping one to experience congruence of thoughts, feelings, and actions. In essence, it is about learning how to attend to the Sacred and self in a manner that allows one to hear and heed the spiritual and emotional needs of others without being subsumed by their pain.
- A process of identifying and developing best practices and competencies for providing spiritual care to diverse clientele.
- A prerequisite for endorsement by most denominations, just as it is a requirement for serving as a military chaplain.
- A requirement for Board Certification by the Association of Professional Chaplains (APC) and other credentialing bodies.
- The standard training process for chaplains in most healthcare systems (See website: http://www.professionalchaplains.org/).

A fundamental principle of CPE is this: What is not well within a chaplain will inevitably surface in the emotions and behaviors of the spiritual caregiver, and if not appropriately addressed and managed, that un-wellness will limit or make hurtful the caregiver's practice of spiritual care. CPE is thus essentially focused on attending to oneself and to the

Sacred as a means of becoming fully present toward others in their pain and loss.

Through my interactions with patients, CPE peers, and hospital staff, I found myself becoming increasingly contemplative regarding my past, present, and future. One afternoon in our didactic time my supervisor defined "addiction" as "a behavior or way of being that we perpetuate even when it does not serve us well." This triggered deeper probing of my thoughts, feelings, and behaviors in the context of my personal history. I wondered: What is there in me that holds me back? What resources is God providing to sort out all of my "baggage"?

CPE was extremely experiential, forcing me to look continually at my inner being with the goal of finding congruence in my personhood. My program was structured to connect my head and heart in the context of relational dynamics.

Here is what was given to and required of me:
- The actual practice of ministry alongside patients, their families, and staff.
- Regular supervision and mentoring by a certified supervisor who had personally experienced the rigors of personal and group accountability.
- Participation in a small group of individuals who covenanted together to provide mutual support and accountability in a safe, confidential manner.
- The sharing with peers of verbatim accounts of interactions with patients with the expectation that my peers would honestly critique my ways of being, listening and speaking.
- Formation of learning objectives congruent with personal needs and competency standards.
- Development of a personal theological and theoretical framework for incorporating specific competencies into my personhood.

Stories are at the heart of CPE. In CPE, the common belief that every person has a story is superseded by the reality that each of us *is* a story. Anton Boisen, pioneer founder of Clinical Pastoral Education, spoke of each individual as being a "Living Human Document." According to his teaching, along with all humankind, each chaplain is constantly being re-written into a Sacred Narrative. Every human interaction is part of a dynamic stream of intersecting lives, all of which influence and are influenced by others.

Every CPE student is invited to lean into the painful process of learning to listen more effectively to where and how the Divine One scripts lives. We listened for the Sacred in patients, we listened for it in peers, and especially, we listened for the movement of the Sacred in places of brokenness, in our own pain and in that of others.

Over the span of three years, I learned to develop meaningful personal goals. My goals became more and more concrete and intentional as my training progressed. One huge shift for me was an awakening to the positive energy of irritants and anger to stimulate and guide personal and systemic transformation. Among other things, developing a theology of anger and befriending it as an informant for justice and mercy became a part of my learning process.

I have a reputation for being "a nice guy," so when a chaplaincy peer told me, "Being nice isn't always nice," I was startled. It took me a while to figure out what he meant. Being nice can be a cover-up. It can mask underlying, unresolved tension.

King David said to his Lord, "Going through the motions doesn't please you; a flawless performance is nothing to you." (Psalm 51:16, *MSG*). Through 30 years of ministry, I strived to please God by giving impeccable service. Indeed, I lived in a manner that many would view as exemplary. I "accomplished" much. Yet, my pastoral persona occasionally masked anger and frustration, representing an incongruence that was symptomatic of a need for healing. Nice on the outside, agitated on the inside!

In striving to please God and others, I often battled feelings of inadequacy. I stuffed anger and silenced my voice when I ought to have tapped into the energy of my anger to become a more effective agent of transformation. In my milieu of frustrated perfectionism, CPE opened some doors of understanding both heavenward and toward myself. I came to understand that saying "No" to evil is a vital component of authentic grace. By listening more deeply for God's voice within the Bible itself, I found myself enthralled and liberated by an awareness that my previously stuffed anger could become holy, healing, and cleansing. The Bible became less of a code book and much more of a case study book; it became much less *prescriptive* of what must be and much more *descriptive* of what happens when God shows up or when the Source of Life is excluded from our world.

When I started CPE, I naively assumed that I had a reasonably good level of maturity, that I had already moved beyond the raw innocence of a novice. Indeed, after I left Japan, I hadn't stopped studying and growing. In addition to my graduate degree in missiology (the theological principles and practices of cross-cultural faith-sharing), I pursued graduate studies in counseling and education. I was confident that I possessed the tools and skill-set of a veteran minister.

However, I was soon flummoxed to see that the "tools in my toolbox" were covered by an accumulation of junk that did not serve me well. As I became increasingly aware of my latent anger and compulsion to avoid conflict, I started learning to be more intentional and more assertive for what is transformative: self-care time, equitable sharing of resources and responsibilities, etcetera. In my new awareness, naiveté about goodness gave way to an expanded appreciation of what is truly holy and sacred.

Like all CPE students, my learning goals and contract contained the following elements:
- **Pastoral Reflection** – contemplation of my personhood in relationship to peers, supervisor, my assigned institution, and the curriculum.
- **Pastoral Identity** – an intentional exploration of personal and pastoral identity issues utilizing various tools of psychology, theology, and culture.
- **Pastoral Competence** – a systematic deepening of pastoral skills with a primary focus on the relational aspects of the human-Divine and human-human experience.

Each of the above goals had a strong theological dimension. I intentionally dug deeper into my personal beliefs and values. My goals compelled me to ask: What is there that informs and holds me when I am living and breathing the daily chaos of the healthcare environment? As I found answers in the Sacred, I grew and paradoxically felt a need for more patience, not less.

I found myself not only reshaping my own attitudes, I wanted to reform the attitudes of others! I often met a variety of startling mindsets that I wanted to "fix." One healthcare administrator stated, "You know, you really don't need all that education to do what you do," indicating a belief that providing a prayer or applying a Scripture verse to a crisis is essentially all that is required to be a chaplain.

Others hinted that chaplains are mostly ministers who have "burned out" or who "failed" as local church pastors. Or, they are soon-to-retire ministers who need a comfortable place to "fill time" until they can collect retirement benefits. Both inside and outside of health care institutions, I met people whose knowledge regarding the training and work of professional chaplains could only be matched by a conviction that the earth is flat.

I learned that pastoring and healthcare chaplaincy ministries are significantly different though there are similarities. When pastoring and teaching I was often asked to help individuals and families during times of crisis. But, the intensity and depth of involvement is different when grief, loss, and pain saturate the work environment *every* day.

Emotional and spiritual resources are stretched to extremes when one is called upon to help deal with 20 different emergency codes, each a life and death situation in one week's time. A young man discharges his gun while cleaning it, nearly killing his pregnant wife; an adolescent has a bullet in his brain as his estranged parents contemplate organ donation; a homeless woman has been raped; a suicidal man enters the hospital lobby, distraught with loneliness after the death of his wife of fifty years; a war veteran has PTSD flashbacks. All are people with needs and wants that pull at heartstrings. The pacing of healthcare chaplaincy mandates that its practitioners be both effective and able to navigate chaos without disintegrating. Integration of beliefs, values, and skills is absolutely essential.

When I entered CPE, I was equipped with "tools" that had been tested and tried in tense moments. However, the disadvantage of long experience is that the container of those tools, my well-seasoned self, needed "a good sorting out." Accumulated memories of my life and ministry had become potential flash points for negative as well as positive connections with patients and their families. CPE provided the opportunity for me to reevaluate and retool. This was done in a unique learning format characterized by peer support.

Part of each day was spent alongside patients and their families. Then the substance of those interactions was brought to my preceptor and my peers. It was a process of action, followed by reflection. I learned that if the action-reflection contemplative processes, typical of CPE, are bypassed, the potential to cause harm is increased.

Indeed, what is not well within a chaplain will inevitably surface in the emotions of the chaplain, and if not appropriately addressed and managed, those feelings may negatively impact effectiveness. When I pastored and taught, I certainly encountered the problems of transference and counter-transference, but rarely to the same extent as I do now as a chaplain. Such challenges are a continual threat as I enter deep into the stories of people's lives. For me, this means that I constantly turn to the transcendent truths that hold and stabilize me in the face of chaos.

During CPE, I discovered that my previous graduate work and experiences in missiology, theology, counseling and education are excellent resources for assisting patients, families and staff with the many questions of life and death that are intrinsic to bedside caregiving. Yet, there were significant gaps in my personal and professional knowledge.

For example: What is the chaplain's ethical and professional responsibility during discussions of brain death and/or organ donation? During medical rounds with the interdisciplinary team, how and when does the chaplain contribute? How does one elicit and process peoples' stories in such a way that freedom of choice is never curtailed? In this process, how does one assess and respond to spiritual pain? Why does offering to say prayers with patients sometimes hinder emotional and spiritual healing? Above all: where, when and how do we encounter the Sacred in our work?

I see the Sacred in the fact that nothing in life is wasted when we give ourselves fully to receive and impart forgiveness and compassion. Though I no longer read, write, and speak Japanese everyday as I once did, I often tap into lessons learned from my cross-cultural history. Today I see patients and families thrust into a new environment in which they see people dressed funny, wearing masks, and speaking unfamiliar jargon. In mastering the Japanese language 40 years ago, I learned that listening always precedes spoken competency, and that attitudes of the heart are more important than flawless pronunciation and grammatical correctness. Perfect speech cannot replace a spirit of loving openness toward others. The same is true in chaplaincy. My past thus intersects with the present in ways that I could not have imagined.

Though my CPE training is behind me now, its lessons continue. During CPE I often turned for encouragement to the poetry and prayers of King David in the Psalms. My heart resonates with his as he goes from lament to worship: "I learned God-worship when my pride was shattered. Heart-shattered lives ready for love don't for a moment escape God's notice" (Psalm 51:17, 18, *MSG*). Like David's encounter with the Divine, the CPE process broke me down and built me up, making my heart more worshipful as I saw how God attends to us in places of profound brokenness. CPE experiences taught me that God heeds my desire to be loved with a powerful rest-giving compassion toward my imperfections.

During David's descent into spiritual brokenness, he cried out, "What you're after is truth from the inside out." He thereafter beseeches, "Enter me, then; conceive a new, true life" (Psalm 51:6, *MSG*). The CPE process embraces the Spirit of this prayer, acknowledging that it is out of places of imperfection and brokenness that the transformed and transformational life emerges. Ministry is thus not so much about being or becoming perfect as it is about being touched by and tapping into transcendent resources that actually work.

As my training progressed, I found that I was discovering and experiencing dimensions of the Sabbath rest on a *daily* basis that helped me to become increasingly a non-anxious, non-judgmental presence both toward others and toward myself. Seeing the Lord of the Sabbath as Lord of All Creation and Restorer of Wellness equips me, as part of that creation, to restfully trust in Ultimate Goodness. I now see the sacred rest permeating Scripture.

Consider how Jesus rose from His rest in a storm-deluged boat to demonstrate His caring heart toward his disciples. From within a place of restfulness, Jesus calms storms and agitated hearts. As I re-embraced the Sabbath and the Incarnate Caring One who rode in that boat, I accepted heaven's antidote for my exhausting production-mentality and my outcome-oriented *modus operandi*. Within the Sabbath promises, I became increasingly able to find God's righteousness intersecting with my brokenness in ways that restored my capacity to stay emotionally present where chaos seemingly reigned. One of the outcomes, for me, of intentional Sabbath awareness throughout the week is that I am now also able to more readily celebrate joyfully what God has done and is doing in and through me.

CPE triggered a kind of Jubilee Celebration. There is new seeing, new hearing, and absolution for my imperfections. In other words, I have tasted a new freedom in ministry. I don't feel quite so compelled now to be the perfect minister because I am now better acquainted with One whose righteousness gives rest and healing when and wherever it is needed. This is something I celebrate.

As I progressed through CPE, my clinical supervisor invited me into his office one morning and extended to me a surprising invitation to join a team of professional chaplains who are assigned to various entities in our region. This invitation unexpectedly altered the trajectory of my ministry. Frequently, I'm awed by how the bits and pieces of my past converge to inform my interactions with patients and staff. It feels as if my temperament, skill-set, and education have coalesced in ways that confirm God's calling of me into this special ministry.

BOARD CERTIFICATION AND GROWTH OPPORTUNITIES

On the day that I was hired as a chaplain, I covenanted in my heart and with my new employer that I would stay on a trajectory of personal and professional growth. For me this meant pursuing Board Certification with the Association of Professional Chaplains.

I found that becoming a Board Certified Chaplain is a lot like learning the Japanese language. You can do either in just 30 minutes or take a longer pathway. Back in the mid-1970s, I struggled to master the subtle nuances of a very complex language. After five hours in class each morning with an interfaith group of missionary peers, I returned home for four more hours of self-flagellation in the evenings as I sought to develop listening, reading, writing and speaking skills. I did this for two years and still struggled. Sixteen years later, I found a newly published book that promised Japanese language proficiency in just 30 minutes. I was amazed and had a conversation with God: "Lord, where was this book when I needed it?" A closer look at the book, of course, revealed that I had been brought down a better path, though a much longer one.

Several websites (you do the searching) promise that one can become a "certified" chaplain in just 30 minutes. Just answer a few simple questions, pay a fee, and in the time it takes to eat a banana split, an elegant certificate and a chaplain's badge are in the mail. Becoming a "chaplain" is that simple, and the benefits are wonderful, including special parking privileges, per one website.

Truly, what makes a chaplain? Sometimes at a patient's bedside, I cry out silently to God, "I don't know what I am doing!" I feel inept and wonder what makes me a credible witness to patients of God's healing presence. If only a 30 minute process could ensure competency and credibility! In fact, answers may be found in a more substantive process of personal and professional growth that is actually never-ending.

Board Certification by credible credentialing bodies such as the Association of Professional Chaplains (APC), National Association of Catholic Chaplains (NACC), and the National Association of Jewish Chaplains (NAJC) indicates that one has demonstrable competencies and an ongoing commitment to growth. The required competencies provide a window that opens up avenues for personal and professional transformation. As one passes through the grid of requirements, one encounters some rough material. But, a sorting out occurs that leaves one feeling energized with an awareness that lifeless stuff has been scraped away and new flesh is emerging.

Right here I want to declare my respect for the many non-certified spiritual caregivers whose personhood and dedication powerfully portrays the presence of the Sacred in their ministry. I am personally acquainted with numerous persons - Protestant, Catholic, Jewish and Muslim - who exhibit exceptional abilities to bring comfort and hope to patients. Some are uniquely able to reach across cultural and religious lines to soothe heartache. These persons are a joy to know and collaborate with. They demonstrate to me that not everyone needs to be certified as a chaplain to provide exemplary spiritual care.

Still, I am convicted that nearly all would-be fulltime chaplains and their employing institutions will benefit from the board certification process. This is because the process of certification highlights best practices and essential competencies, along with the importance of practical theological integration.

At its core the process asks: Are we actively engaging in processes of transformation so that our competencies as professional chaplains reflect a commitment to experiencing growth and wholeness in the presence and power of the Sacred? Are we becoming more and more trustworthy in our caregiving?

Every healthcare professional goes through rigorous processes of testing, credentialing, and continuing education. It is no different for chaplains. Certification provides avenues for ongoing growth and accountability similar to those required for other healthcare providers. It also brings credibility to chaplains as members of interdisciplinary care teams.

Here is what is involved in a professional chaplain's preparation for Board Certification:

- A Master of Divinity Degree (MDiv) or its equivalent – three years of full time education in theology, spirituality, religion and culture at an accredited university.
- Four units of Clinical Pastoral Education – a minimum of one year of full time classroom and clinical studies with a peer group under the supervision of a credentialed clinical pastoral educator. (A residency provides four units of Clinical Pastoral Education).
- Denominational endorsement and credentialing – a sometimes lengthy process that seeks to ensure that chaplains have beliefs, values, and relational connections that can hold and sustain them through stressful circumstances.
- Two thousand hours of chaplaincy employment after completing four units of Clinical Pastoral Education.
- Evidence of specific competencies.
- Application with a portfolio of documentation to the Association of Profession Chaplains or a similar accrediting body, and then an appearance before a panel of Board Certified Chaplains who have reviewed the applicant's personal and professional development and his/her commitment to ethical and professional standards of spiritual care. (See www.professionalchaplains.org and www.acpe.edu).

CERTIFICATION AND CREDIBILITY

In an era of increased competiveness for healthcare dollars, hospitals are increasingly looking for skilled professionals in all areas of patient care. Part of this is driven by the "best practice standards" and expectations of hospital regulatory and accrediting agencies. Chaplains are caught in this specialization current. It is very rare now to find a job posting for a full time chaplaincy position that does not require both denominational endorsement and Board Certification by a recognized certifying organization.

There are reasons for this. Professional chaplains are known to directly impact a hospital's financial bottom line in some specific ways:

- Professional chaplains improve staff retention. Administrators increasingly see trained chaplains as contributors not only to patient wellness, but as enhancers of staff morale. By diffusing staff angst and stress through post-event interventions, staff turnover rates and expensive recruitment costs are reduced.
- Staff chaplains who network with community clergy create loyal patrons. When multiple entities are vying for potential patients, community clergy are more inclined to direct their parishioners to the facility where they believe he/she will receive the best, most holistic care, inclusive of respect for diverse spiritual and religious practices.
- Professional chaplains are trained to work with risk management staff in volatile, potentially litigious situations in ways that respect institutional priorities while advocating for patient rights. Avoidance of just one major lawsuit more than covers the annual costs of staffing a hospital with professionally equipped spiritual care providers.

While I was yet in training, an administrator told me that I had just personally saved the hospital from a lengthy litigious process the previous week. At the bedside of a dying patient, I had experienced an angry doctor, an angry family, and a nursing staff with their professional loyalties being stretched to a near breaking point. The situation also involved religious and spiritual beliefs. My intentions that night were not about protecting the hospital from a lawsuit, but that outcome was a direct result of my listening to anger, and recommending a few simple changes in how the medical team was communicating with the family. My interventions dealt with staff morale, collaboration with community clergy, and ethical and legal considerations – all elements of patient-centered care as it impacts a hospital's bottom line.

Though motivations for hiring skilled chaplains are not always altruistic, this trend toward professionalization of spiritual care provides opportunities for men and women who have professional credibility. Increasingly this means Board Certification.

CERTIFICATION AND A CODE OF ETHICS

Each chaplaincy certifying body espouses a code of ethics that reflects values which guide its membership. Early in my CPE training, I read this in the APC Code of Ethics: "Members shall affirm the religious and spiritual freedom of all persons and refrain from imposing doctrinal positions or spiritual practices on persons whom they encounter in their professional role as chaplains." At first glance, I wondered: does this curtail religious zeal? One word in this statement intersects with one of my deeply held core values – freedom. My own quest into the faith of my ancestors informs me that coercion in any form is Biblically incongruous with the character of the God and the church that I represent. The same God who knew in advance that Adam's free choice would result in indescribably profound pain to Himself still upheld Adam's capacity to choose wrongly as a prerequisite for authentic loving.

A close perusal of the above ethics statement makes it clear that members are, in fact, NOT being asked to validate every religious belief that floats across the horizon. Nor are they being asked to abandon deeply held personal convictions. Rather, each chaplain is asked to honor every person's right to follow the dictates of his or her own conscience. This innate freedom mandates that chaplains learn when and how to listen and when and how to speak. I believe that this is congruent with the values of most conservatives and liberals (or most others in the religious spectrum). One may be conservative in one's own values and beliefs while being liberal in kindness toward all.

Above all, I have experienced the Code of Ethics as a summons to be sensitive toward the Sacred. In the certification process, the required 29 competencies become an expression of this calling. One of my colleagues, a devout Christian jail chaplain, was recently quizzed regarding how he "brings" Christ to inmates." He said, "I do not 'bring' Christ. I believe that Christ is already there – there before I come, and there after I leave." Such a stance acknowledges personal limitations and affirms the power of God to transcend any human tendency or capacity to indoctrinate or "guide" a person. While it leaves the results of our presence in God's care, it also affirms the presence of God in places that are seemingly void of God's Spirit. I find this perspective to be liberating. It sets me free from performance anxieties related to a need to "fix" something. The outcome is not dependent on me. Simply knowing that God has a high regard toward each of His children opens my heart more widely to sacred possibilities.

During my CPE training and board certification process, I was surrounded by peers and preceptors who modeled these values, never denigrating my spiritual journey. In choice-honoring ways, they prompted me to explore more deeply what there is within my personal beliefs and values that can hold me in the midst of chaotic circumstances. This was fundamental to my development as a chaplain and has made it possible for me to avoid burnout. This has been to my benefit, and I believe it has helped others too.

MORE THAN A CASUAL COMMITMENT

In addition to examining and agreeing to adhere to a Code of Ethics, APC applicants are asked to submit a portfolio of materials and then appear before a panel of certified peers who have reviewed all materials and identified talking points for further growth. Typically the packet represents five to six years of education and training beyond one's bachelors degree. The APC website has detailed information regarding application content and deadlines for submission. Note that in certain instances the APC grants equivalencies for Clinical Pastoral Education and graduate studies that have not led to a Master of Divinity degree.

Each applicant is required to provide documented evidence that he/she is self-aware and competent in 29 specific areas. My colleagues in most critical care areas of healthcare have at least that demanding of a process – often much more. Thus, I don't think it is too much to ask of the chaplain discipline. By pursuing personal and professional growth for ourselves as chaplains, we demonstrate respect for those who are on parallel professional trajectories. As others give their best to their patients and colleagues, we want to do likewise.

Colleagues tell me that certification is not so much about complete mastery of competencies as it is about taking responsibility to grow in self-awareness with a solid commitment to claim one's full potential as a well-integrated servant of the Sacred. The peer review aids self-discovery. Interviewers look for ongoing integration. The panel probes and prods to identify strengths as well as growth areas. It is grueling. Though a person may be denied immediate membership in the APC, denial is not the panel's intent. Integrative growth is the objective.

Following certification, members must complete a minimum of 50 hours of continuing education annually to maintain membership, and must undergo a peer review process every five years. Each Board Certified Chaplain is required to pursue specific personal and professional growth objectives just as he/she did while in Clinical Pastoral Education. Each denominational endorser may have similar processes of accountability.

In all this, one thing is clear. Just as my many years studying the Japanese language and culture were rewarded by precious lifelong friendships, all the time spent in quest of personal growth and professional excellence brings surprises of profound grace as patients, their families and staff see how much we care. For me, this is certainly worth more than a casual commitment.

A Model for Community-wide Spiritual Care

When The Reverend Wes McIntyre, my CPE supervisor/teacher, conveyed a job offer to me from Tri-Cities Chaplaincy (also known as The Chaplaincy), I joined a unique organization. In 1971, The Reverend John Moody was a local clergyman who had observed that during a medical crisis, patients and their families often need spiritual care that is conversant with the complexities of the healthcare environment and is simultaneously honoring of diverse needs, wishes and choices. So, he spoke with area churches and launched an initiative to bring professional chaplaincy training to the region.

Today, in addition to training chaplains in a program accredited by the Department of Education, The Chaplaincy offers a full range of services that reflect its heritage. In addition to providing chaplains at hospitals, it attends to the physical, emotional, and spiritual needs of hospice patients in homes, diverse care facilities, and a dedicated Hospice House; licensed bereavement counselors offer personal and group support for men, women, and children; another team of licensed mental health therapists provides Medical Family Therapy, a counseling approach that helps families find a new equilibrium after a catastrophic or chronic diagnosis has disrupted a family system. Additionally it contracts to provide professional chaplaincy services to both correctional institutions and hospitals.

As a newly hired chaplain, I was assigned to Kadlec Regional Medical Center, the flagship of The Chaplaincy's contracting partners. I become one of a team of caregivers committed to making our community a better place for all.

Today, all of The Chaplaincy's chaplains are either board certified, seeking board certification, or have a type of licensure equivalency. The group includes persons with backgrounds in nursing, education, social work, marriage and family therapy, or pulpit ministries with related degrees and licenses. Each has made clinical pastoral education part of their journey into chaplaincy.

The Chaplaincy is unique in that all of its chaplains are not only clinically educated, they are also *cross-trained, screened and oriented to serve at multiple, otherwise unrelated sites.* This means that a hospital or hospice chaplain, or emergency service chaplain may go many directions when on-call at night – to any of several hospitals, or to a hospice patient's bedside at his home or in a facility. Likewise, Emergency Service Chaplains, Cancer Center chaplains, hospital chaplains, and hospice chaplains can converge at a hospital when there is a Mass Critical Incident such as the crash of a fully loaded school bus.

The team's diverse areas of expertise are available across the spectrum of human life throughout the community. The team delivers specialty services such as Critical Incident Stress Management debriefings whenever needed following traumatizing events. These services are delivered in hospitals, businesses, schools, and other places where people's lives have been changed by an upsetting loss or death.

CITYWIDE SPIRITUAL CARE HANDOFFS

How does this work in a complex social milieu? Consider what happens when a car spins out of control on the interstate that passes through Tri-Cities. Bill, an Emergency Services chaplain, is at the accident scene alongside fire crews and highway patrol. He calls me at Kadlec, saying. "No fatalities, but we've got a man headed your direction... maybe a stroke... intubated... I'm with the family now... We should be there not long after the ambulance..."

Seconds later, I hear an overhead announcement: "Stroke Team Activation, Emergency Department, Room 18." Soon thereafter, Bill hands off care of the family to me at the entrance to the ED's treatment room. I give the family a brief glimpse of the convergence of clinical support, then take them to a quiet room where I assess their needs and wishes, provide them with access to phones, pray with them at their request, and then contact Marvin, their pastor. During the evolving crisis, I periodically update the family with information from Room 18 where the patient is being stabilized. Later I hand over care to Cheryl, another staff chaplain, who tracks the patient's progress from ED to the CT Lab, and then to the Intensive Care Unit. During this process a brain tumor is identified.

There are multiple interactions with the family on subsequent days during interdisciplinary morning rounds, Family Care Conferences, and drop-in visits to the family. Care options point toward either life-altering aggressive treatment at Tri-Cities Cancer Center or comfort care with Hospice at The Chaplaincy. At each of these sites a professional chaplain is present to receive a hand-off for emotional and spiritual care.

As the crisis progresses, the patient becomes increasingly restless and agitated. A family member tells the chaplain that the patient has a son with whom he has not spoken in many years. That son is now in jail. After speaking with the patient's spouse and obtaining her consent, I call the jail chaplain. This results in an ancient estrangement being healed. The patient's face relaxes and he rests as transfer plans to Hospice House are finalized. When he arrives at Hospice at The Chaplaincy, Paul, a hospice chaplain, welcomes him and accompanies him in his ongoing journey. One week later the patient dies with his family, pastor, and chaplain alongside. From the site of his fender bender to the time of his death he and his family have had immediate access to spiritual and religious support at *every* transitional point and also in between.

INTERDISCIPLINARY COLLABORATION

This quest for seamless spiritual care is a collaborative process citywide and within institutions. For example, during a patient's coronary artery bypass surgery at Kadlec, when the silence of extended waiting exacerbates anxiety, chaplains deliver periodic progress reports from the operating room team to family members. For such patients and their families, pre-op, post-op and intermediate visits by a chaplain occur according to protocols collaboratively developed with an interdisciplinary team.

After the patient is transferred from the OR to the Intensive Care Unit, chaplains remain connected to the patient through participation in morning rounds. In the midst of clinical reports, a chaplain may be asked to help arrange a family care conference involving the intensivist, bedside nurse, social worker, and discharge planner to clarify aspects of a care plan. At such times the chaplain may function as an advocate for patient and/or family. If an ethical, cultural, or religious dilemma emerges, the chaplain will help facilitate an on-site ethical discernment process and will collaborate with the family's clergy for guidance.

Dialing Up Self-care

The on-call system maintained by this group of chaplains also effectively enables chaplains to avoid "pager burnout." Rather than the typical pattern of an institution's on-call responsibilities descending on only a few persons, no chaplain at any of The Chaplaincy's partnering institutions carries a pager more than three or four nights a month. While on-call, each chaplain covers not only his/her own assigned institution but also those of his/her peers. The off–call chaplains have the opportunity to rest more freely, knowing that their institution's spiritual care is in the hands of a trained colleague who will network with community clergy to deliver spiritual care that honors each recipient's needs and wishes.

In order to manage the rigors of caregiving, the citywide chaplaincy team meets once a week for 90 minutes. In this circle of mutual support, chaplains share a covenant of personal and professional accountability, providing each other with opportunities to diffuse stress and maintain personal well-being.

The group maps its core values and defines itself with these words: "We are a collaborative, committed, accountable community that speaks the truth in love, that cares for one another through emotional, spiritual and physical transitions, and where tensions, exhaustion and exhilaration are shared and understood and held in supportive space. We are miners/mortals who engage the deep stories of life and meaning that connect with the Sacred Story." The quest for wellness is thus a shared journey. It is a matter of community.

HITTING THE EMOTIONAL WALL

It was a nightmarish situation. My wife and I had crossed multiple time zones to land in Tokyo, Japan for a short holiday. Our jet-lagged arrival at the hotel in the middle of the night brought sweet slumber. After awakening in the morning, we consulted briefly with the concierge and set out to explore. We wandered leisurely through bustling streets for several kilometers to a high-rising *depaato* (department store). After so many years away, it felt natural and wonderful to bask in the sounds and smells of nostalgia, being back in Japan where I had spent so many formative years of my young adulthood. Japanese speech flowed freely from my lips – totally unlike my first landing in Japan forty years earlier. It felt good to be back in my adopted homeland.

Then I glanced down at my trousers and realized that somehow they were ripped in an unsightly way. Briefly I spoke with Bonnie, asking, "Do you mind if I go back to the hotel and change?" She affirmed the wisdom of this.

So, I dashed down the store escalators, back to ground level, quick-paced back to our hotel room where I hastily donned a different pair of slacks. Without pausing, I deescalated to the lobby, waved to a grinning concierge, and plunged back out onto the teaming sidewalks. Ten, fifteen minutes later, I paused at an intersection, and glanced up and around. And then down, and realized that I was wearing pajama bottoms. Furthermore, I realized that I had taken a wrong turn and was lost.

Though I spoke fluent Japanese to passing strangers, I couldn't remember the name of our hotel or the name of the department store where I had left my wife.

However, I did know her name and cell phone number. So, I reached for my cell phone to call her. Oops! No phone. It was clipped to my torn trousers back in the hotel room.

Frustrated and embarrassed, I took a deep breath and strategized. I'll take a taxi to her, I thought. She must be getting worried. As I contemplated how to instruct the driver to take me to a place with a name that I did not remember, I reached for my billfold to see if I had enough *yen*. It was then that I realized that my yang was out of sync with my yen. No wallet! It too was with my former trousers. More and more worried, I wondered, how in God's creation did I get so turned around and so muddled? What a mulish nightmare! (Yes, it really was all a nightmare – a *very* bad dream from which I awakened covered in sweat.)

People sometimes ask me if I dream in Japanese. Yes, dreams and nightmares occasionally alert me regarding the undercurrents of life, revealing unspoken and unspeakable anxieties. For example, I don't want to struggle with the kind of memory issues that now assault my aging parents. I don't want to fail to be present when my wife needs me. I don't want to look back over my life and feel that I've just been a strange stranger among strangers, that I've failed others and myself. I yearn for connectedness that transcends all fears. And no matter how old I am, I want to *enjoy* life, tapping into resources that help navigate through the realities of human brokenness.

Today I am a professional chaplain by God's design and part of a supportive community. Though I am sometimes flummoxed by the mysteries of the mind, heart, and spirit, I awaken each day to the truth that I am in a good place, loved by a lovable God, and attired in hope that transcends torn slacks and nightmarish pajamas. And at the end of the day, I am at peace.

Chapter 4

CREATING SPACE TO RETREAT (AND ADVANCE)

AWAKENING TO SNAPSHOTS OF GLORY

High in the mountains of western Japan is a rustic lakeside cabin where I sometimes rested and rejuvenated between exhausting stints of busyness in congested cities. Year-round snow glistened on distant peaks, sending its frigid melt-off down canyons into deep waters. For me, Lake Nojiri was a soul-nurturing sanctuary away from city stresses.

During my retreats, I discovered an amazing phenomenon. If I awakened early and rowed out from shore at dawn before the heat of the day, I could see mirror images of spectacular peaks reflecting on glassy water. Light and shadows danced across pristine liquid as the sun ascended. Time and again I experienced snapshots of glory.

However, some days I clung to the comfort of bed, letting the sun arise before me. On those days, I missed the morning reflection. By the time I awakened, the rising sun cast its heat upon the waters. Winds came down from the mountains, putting feathered white caps on wave tops. Powerboats and jet skis further stirred the water, spewing out noise across the landscape. Gone was the glorious double blessing of the horizon until evening's coolness came.

The Native American Traditional Code of Ethics starts with these words: "Each morning upon rising, and each evening before sleeping, give thanks for the life within you and for all life, for the good things the Creator has given you and for the opportunity to grow a little more each day. Consider your thoughts and actions of the past day and seek for the courage and strength to be a better person. Seek the things that will benefit others." What rocks my little boat is the realization that life is a lake of opportunities. If we miss the morning calm, we can yet claim the breeze off the mountains to fill our sails and propel us where powerboats cannot go on empty tanks. Whether it is early, late, or in between, we may experience the profound joy of discovery.

(See *www.sapphyr.net/natam/nacodeethics.htm* for the complete Native American Code of Ethics).

HOW ABOUT THOSE PEACH SEEDS?

I believe that finding time and means to decompress is vital for sustaining body, mind, and spirit when caught up in the frenetic pace of caregiving. Some people decompress on the face of a granite wall, inserting fingers and toes into narrow cracks and fissures. Others release their stress underneath zillions of gallons of water as fish (and maybe some sharks) swim with them across coral reefs. Still others unload the weight of their being by creating silky illusions of insects on fishhooks. Ancient Chinese artisans carved boats and birds and emperors on cherry pits and peach seeds. But, how do you find relief from life's pressures when you don't have access to a rock wall, coral reefs, streams, or cherry pits and peach seeds?

Though many find participation in religious activities and programs to be restorative, others do not. When Grandma is deathly ill, and her family is waiting for a hospice intake nurse to come and talk with them, it is hard for them to be in a church, synagogue, or temple with others whose minds might be on a golf course or an upcoming ball game. A respiratory therapist or nurse who has been awake all night tending to a critical patient may not be able to stay awake through an 11 o'clock sermon. The healthcare environment cries out for soul-nurturing support that is congruent with the needs of people whose emotional stresses and body clocks are out of sync with "normal" life.

Experience tells us that, if not cared for, the cumulative impact of grief after grief and crisis after crisis can cause breakdowns in effective functioning within both institutions and individuals. Chaplains too get tired.

Since no person can be in all places at all times for all people, and since no amount of religious programming will meet every need, it is important to ask, what is manageable?

Can a hospital with a finite number of staff chaplains realistically offer daily morning and evening chapel services while the Emergency Department and Intensive Care Unit are announcing Code Blues overhead? Not likely! So, how can an institution that is awake around the clock provide stress release opportunities for its employees without multiplying pep talks and scheduling myriad debriefings? Stresses can be eased by creatively providing silent, self-paced retreats in a safe neutral environment.

The chapel is potentially a hospital's greatest self-care resource. In times of personal crisis when feeling overwhelmed by emotional, physical, and spiritual exhaustion, the chapel provides a place not far from the hectic pace of constant *doing,* enabling the occupier of the space to simply *be.* Be relaxed, be rested, and be restored.

A chapel is different from a church, mosque, synagogue or meeting place. It is intended to be a safe, neutral zone for anyone and everyone to quietly explore the inner resources of the soul regardless of religious heritage. Some, in fact, might say that it's mighty like a fishing hole! In quiet contemplation, the heart may be opened to perceive the Divine working in diverse ways to bring about healing of the body, mind, and spirit.

STRESS-RELEASING SELF-PACED RETREATS

From time to time, our chaplain team sponsors silent, self-paced "retreats" in the chapel that provide unique opportunities and resources for personal rejuvenation and the revitalization of community. These are accessible around the clock and do not require the presence of a homiletician or liturgical expert. During these walk-through meditations, signage invites visitors to sit for a while in front of a series of simple contemplation stations, each with visual triggers to assist the viewer in a journey toward inner tranquility. Sensory symbols such as water and light are used to help process feelings, thoughts, and related matters of faith. Each stopping place is equipped with a carefully crafted script that evokes self-assessment, contemplation of the Sacred, and a relinquishment of anxieties. Retreats are designed to bring hope where there is despair, ease where there is dis-*ease,* and even a nap where there is exhaustion.

No symbol of the onward journey is more utilized than our chapel's rocking chair. Have you ever rocked facing backward in a rocking chair? Probably not since you were an infant in your parents' arms! As an adolescent and teenager I often safely straddled straight-backed dining chairs in the wrong direction, but not rocking chairs. I learned early in my childhood that facing backward in a rocking chair is not such a healthy idea. In rocking chairs, balance remains better with forward orientation. The rocking chair is thus a metaphor for life's choices. It serves to re-orient us from a backward-looking passive acceptance of life's offerings toward an active rest as we face forward. Stress is released as we rock along with gentle movements of faith.

As you continue reading *A Bamboo Grove for the Soul,* imagine that you are alone with your personal needs in a sacred space. Let the *italicized* script and artistry of each page guide you at your own pace from experience to experience as if you were actually in a chapel, trekking from scene to scene.

Each walk-through retreat is developed thematically with four or more mediation stations in a recommended sequence. However, readers are encouraged to be selective, embracing all, some, or none. Above all, my hope is that readers will find their own creative juices stimulated to develop new ways of interacting with the spiritual needs of their patrons. One may choose to use an entire sequence, modifying language along the way. Or one may choose to create just one or two stopping places. By periodically altering our approach, we allow new worshipful energy to awaken.

Some of the retreats are distinctly Christian in nature, reflecting reoccurring requests of hospital patronage. Others have a more inter-religious flavor. Retreats are nuanced to the needs and requests of staff and visitors. For example, you will find several Lent and Easter meditation experiences. You will also find "Cracking the Funny Bone," a walk-through meditation retreat that focuses on the healing properties of laughter.

Please be aware that these scripts have the two dimensional limitations of paper (or an e-book screen). But, imagination is powerful. Let it carry you beyond finite restraints into the unparalleled multi-dimensional realm of the Infinite One, into that space that is above and beyond the walls of hospital chapels.

THE BRIDGE TO WELLNESS

Station 1: Light and Shadows

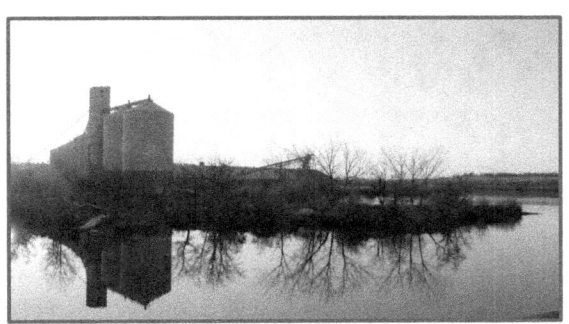

Take time for reflection. Any regrets in your life? How do you rise above the turbulent undercurrents of the "would've, could've, should've" dynamics of broken promises and resolutions? Contemplate:

- *Have you burned some bridges behind you? If so, why?*
- *What meaning and purpose upholds you now as you face the future? Can you identify something that sustains you?*
- *Consider the ancient story of a broken young man:*

> *"When he came to his senses, he said, '...I will set out and go back to my father and say to him: Father, I have sinned against heaven and against you. I am no longer worthy to be called your son; make me like one of your hired servants.' So he got up and went to his father...While he was still a long way off, his father saw him and was filled with compassion for him; he ran to his son, threw his arms around him and kissed him" (Luke 15:11-20, NIV).*

- *How does the spirit of forgiveness transport you beyond wallowing in self-blame and guilt?*
- *Prayerfully identify a painful memory for which you desire healing, then aim a prayer heavenward, trusting that all of heaven is reaching out to receive you with an open heart. When you feel ready, quietly move to the next station.*

Station 2: Reflections and Relationships

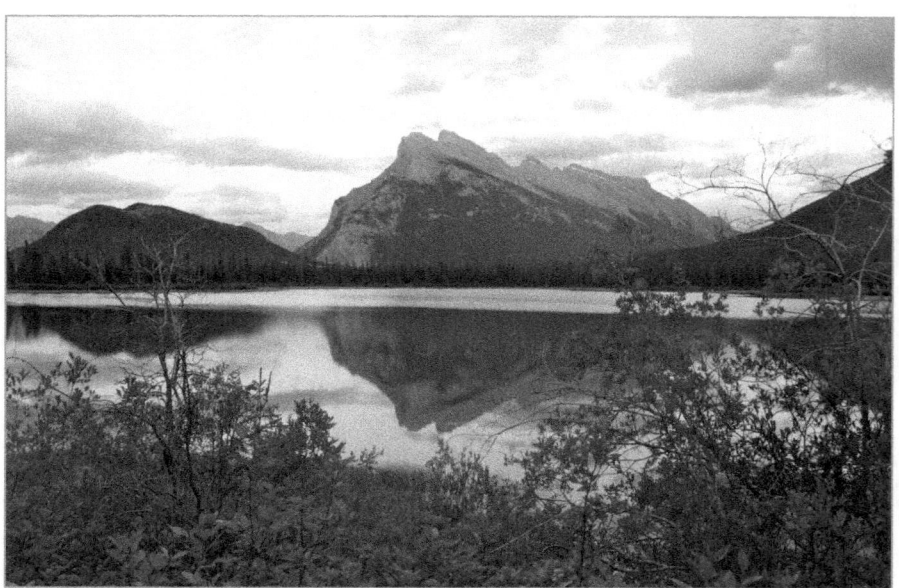

Life's most chaotic moments are often times of life review. As you reflect on your past while seeking a future, do you sometimes feel torn by turbulent circumstances, part of you reaching for a crumbling shore and part of you stretching for an elusive life ring as it passes by? Sometimes we get stretched between life's realities and elusive hopes. In those moments, to what or to whom do you cling? Contemplate:

- *No one crosses a bridge without some measure of trust in the designer and the construction crew. What/who is in your heart today?*
- *Bridges have many parts: footings, girders, trusses, cables, railings, and etcetera. Who/what is the focus of your faith?*
- *What do you need in order to feel at peace internally as you navigate across the deep, relentless currents of change?*
- *Solomon, an ancient king, said of God, "He has planted eternity in the human heart" (Ecclesiastes 3:11, NLT) so that they might seek the Divine. Do you believe that the far shore is there even when you can't see it?*
- *Spend a few moments checking your internal compass, and then prayerfully send up some "flare prayers" for further guidance. When you are ready, move to the next station.*

Station 3: Brokenness and Blessedness

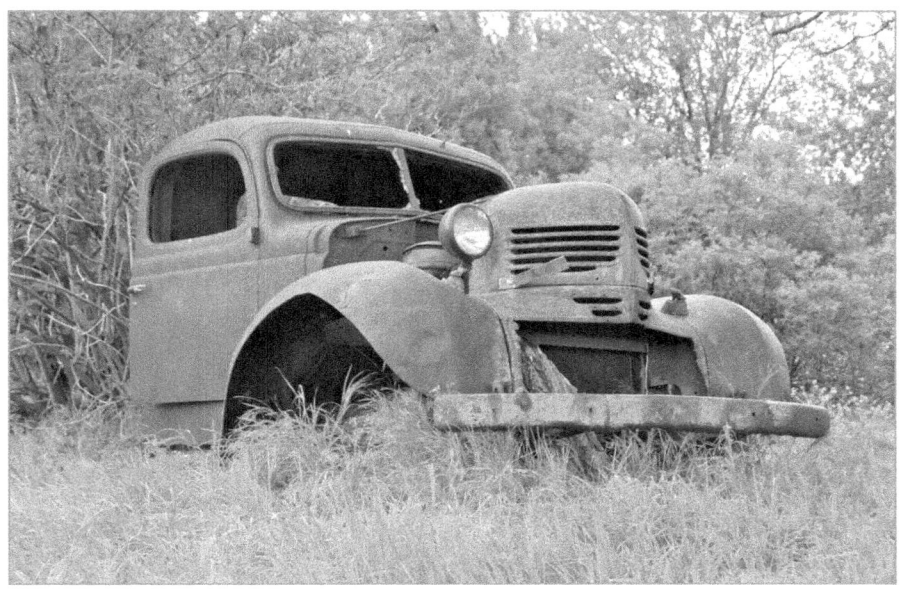

When an artery of the heart is blocked or deteriorates, it is said that the body compensates for a while by creating alternative avenues for blood to flow to blood-starved areas. Indeed, alongside the brokenness of life there is a blessedness that carries us through difficulties. Truly the soul grows through loss. Contemplate:

- In hindsight, can you identify moments when you felt broken and abandoned like an old car, but were in fact surrounded by divine graciousness? How have those experiences extended and expanded the horizons of your life?
- Pause to prayerfully count your blessings. Let the brokenness of the past be cleansed away and then move forward in a newness of being.
- Today allow yourself to be a child again taking baby steps in the grand adventure of life. Seek now the next resting place.

Station 4: Stretching and Serving

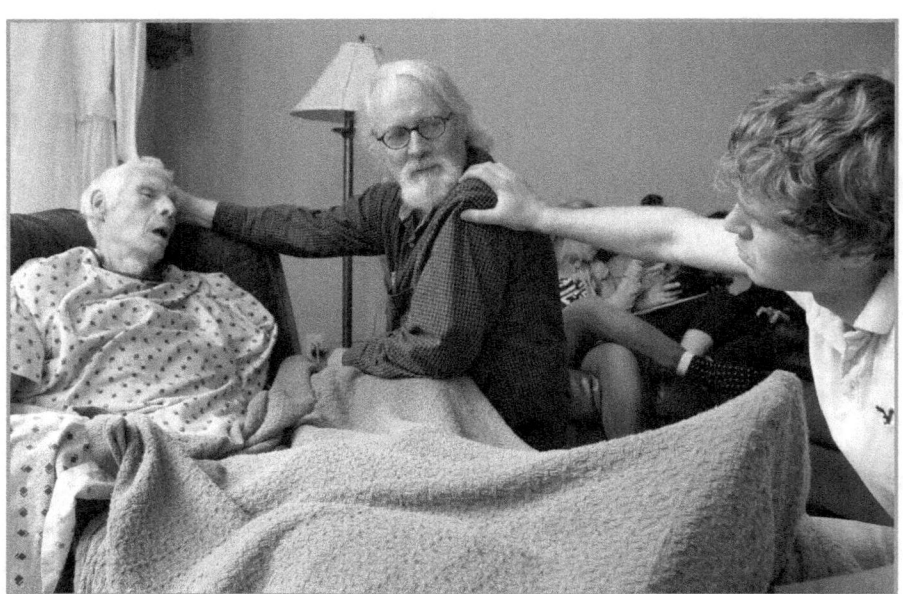

The difference between an estate and a legacy is the difference between what is in one's bank account and what endures in the heart of those we love after we die. An estate is about money, property, insurance and possessions, whereas a legacy is about memories, hopes and aspirations. In the grand scheme of life **each individual is a bridge to the next generation.** Contemplate:

- What is your legacy? Sacred Writings declare, "There are three things that last forever – faith, hope and love. But, the greatest of these is love." Is this your legacy?
- How does your way of being with people create a pathway for them across troublesome places?
- Today stretch out your body, mind and spirit to span the space between heaven and earth. Prayerfully lay claim to the resources of heaven. With muscles of grace, will you become a bridge of love "over troubled water"?
- When you've stretched far and your muscles falter, let go and let the Highest Power hold you.
- Then, when you are ready to re-engage with the world, go in peace and the power of faith, hope and love.

CRACKING THE FUNNY BONE

It's an old joke. Perhaps you've heard it. A woman had two chickens. One got sick so she made chicken soup out of the healthy one to help the sick one get better. Around the world each day caregivers come alongside hurting men, women and children for whom chicken soup alone is not enough for wellness. What helps? When the cure feels as bad as the disease, sometimes a little laughter can change our perspective.

We are given two legs upon which to walk, one called "reality" and the other called "hope." Humor becomes the sacred therapist that aligns these legs to keep them moving toward wellness. As we trek along our legs may be pulled again and again, so much so that we become taller and our heads bump against silver linings in cloudy skies.

So, put your nose to the grindstone, your shoulder to the wheel, your hand on the plow, your foot on the pedal, and your eyes on the stars! (Be careful if you're in a cow pasture.) Now, try to do something important. Anything! The contortions of our dreams are all in the quest of a silver lining. Humor helps unscramble our legs; it sorts out realities and aspirations in such a way that the impossible becomes possible, and our faith is fulfilled.

Reinhold Niebuhr once observed that humor and faith are part of the same journey. Humor looks at life's immediate questions of life and breath while faith looks for ultimate meaning and purpose. Humor is often a prelude into sacred time and space, leading to prayer and praise.

So, heed the signs as you cruise through our chapel. When you hit a speed bump, will you see stars, hit a silver lining, or simply go "ouch"? Proceed at your own pace (and risk).

Catapult 1: Take a Breather!

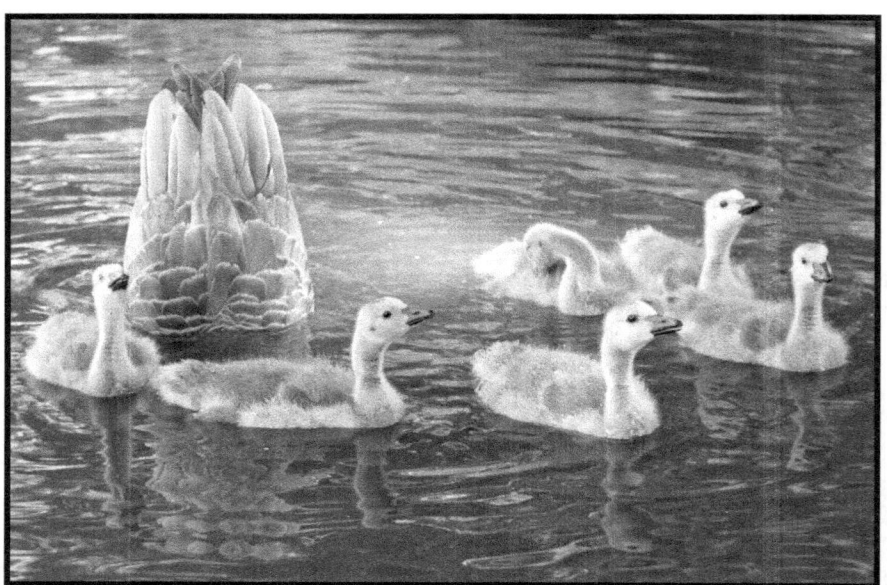

Imagine that you are a mama duck with lots of responsibilities for the welfare of others. Listen to the water flowing.

- *What do you need today?*
- *Put your head down and your tail in the air.*
- *Say a prayer and let the world swirl around you.*
- *Float wherever your spirit takes you.*
- *When you are ready to come up for air, paddle to the next station.*

Catapult 2: Roll with the Punch Line

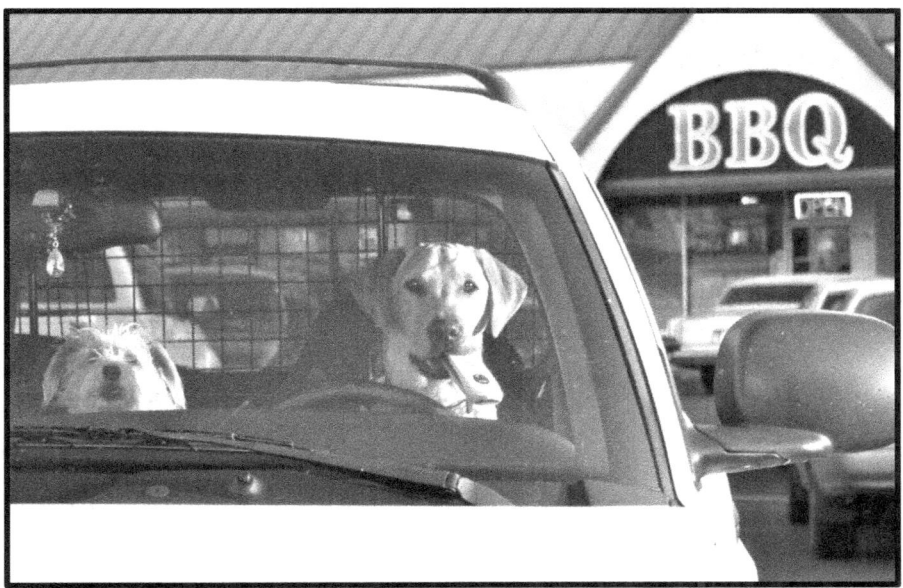

Photo by Bonnie Oneonta-Becraft

King Solomon said, "A joyful heart is good medicine, but a broken spirit dries up the bones" (Proverbs 17:22, HCSB). Except for the pain associated with sidesplitting laughter or the occasional embarrassment (or bladder reaction) of an uncontrolled guffaw, humor helps us emotionally, physically, and spiritually.

- *Contemplate this photo of two dogs out on the town. How does it speak to you?*
- *Recall a time when you experienced a deep belly laugh. In that moment, how did the sacred touch your humanity?*
- *What helps you navigate stressful times? Any sacred resources?*
- *After you've identified a healing point of laughter, embrace the future and move to the next station.*

Catapult 3: Find the Goose in the Noose

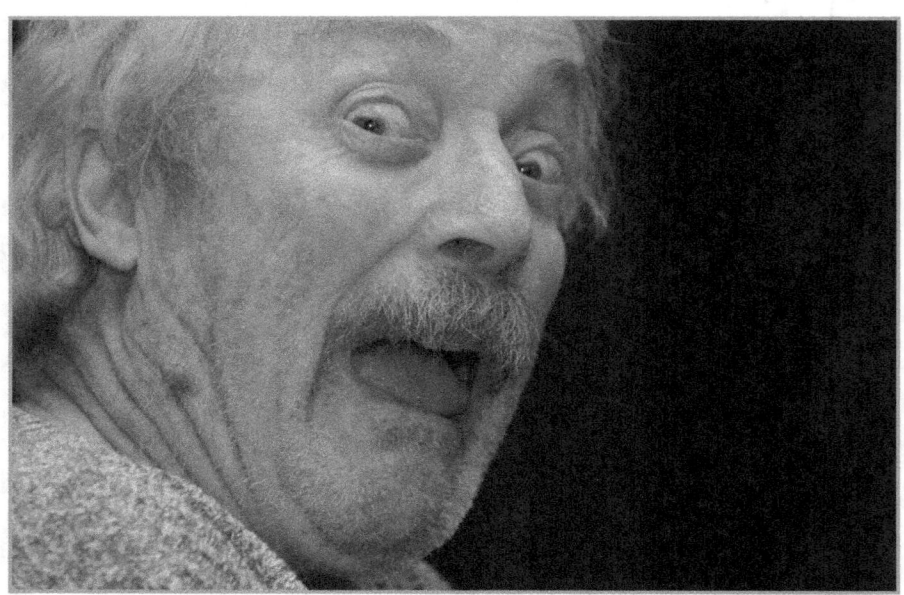

What does it mean to be living each day with knowledge of your mortality? Can you laugh at death? Below is a modern sonnet inspired by John Donne, an English poet, satirist, and cleric of the early 17th century. Donne wrote, "Death be not proud, though some have called thee Mighty and dreadfull, for, thou art not soe...." In modern lingo, think now of death as a goose:

Mighty? It is not so!
You crow like a goose
with your neck in a noose
and are bound for woe.
O Bully, you have met your foe.
Sing now the blues,
for we've got news.
Death will die and fear will go.
O Thug, the death that you willed
is now a ring in your nose
since the Lord forever arose
to sow good in the tomb that you tilled.
Those whose life you spilled

will rise with faith unshaken
as from sleep they awaken
forever freed from the dungeon you built.
Death is but a snore that will be no more.

Today, we grapple with the stark realities of daily decay while believing in ultimate transcendence. With one foot on earth and the other in heaven, we do the "splits," stretching ourselves in a journey of discovery. Earthly humor expands our souls. Prayer becomes an exclamation mark in the comedic journey of our lives. Allow time now for conversation between your heart and the Divine:

- *What might you say to the Divine that would cause laughter in heaven?*
- *What might God say that would bring joy to your heart?*
- *When you are done, take a smile with you back into the comedic stream of life.*

Vessels of Hope and Healing

Station 1: The Ink Pot and the Parchment

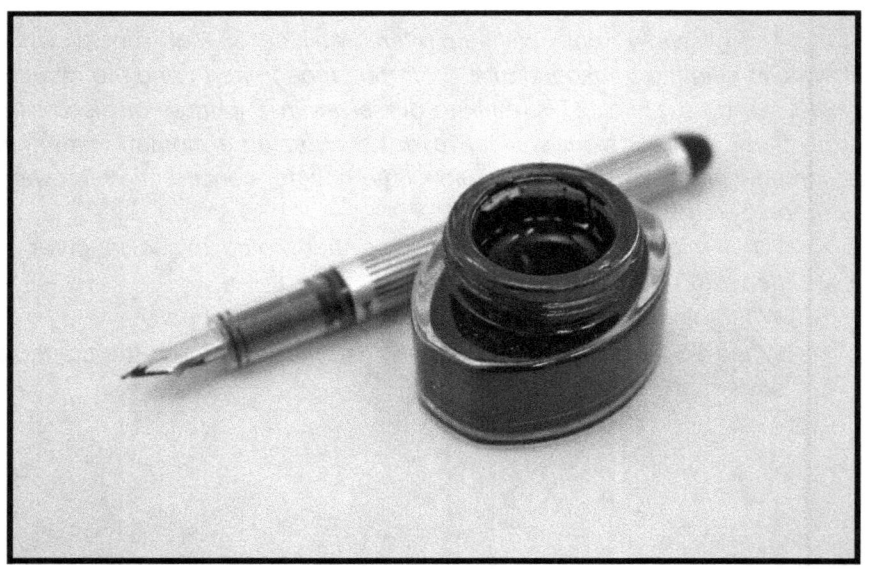

It is often said, "Everyone has a story." But, perhaps it is more accurate to say, "Everyone *is* a story" – a story that is continuously moving toward a mysterious conclusion. *Consider these words: Let us keep "fixing our eyes on Jesus, the author and perfecter of faith, who for the joy set before Him endured the cross, despising the shame, and has sat down at the right hand of the throne of God" (Hebrews 12:2, NASB).*

- *Quietly and prayerfully imagine that the Divine Writer is extending his hand toward you, touching you with his pen. Let yourself feel the gentleness of heaven's Spirit-breath as the sacred hand moves boldly and gently across your heart.*
- *As you breathe out, release your anxieties.*
- *As you breathe in, savor the fragrance of hope and healing.*
- *Rest and relax and let your story be written. (Should we say, "Re-written"?)*
- *When your heart yearns for more, proceed to the next station.*

Station 2: The Scarred Vessels and the Potpourri

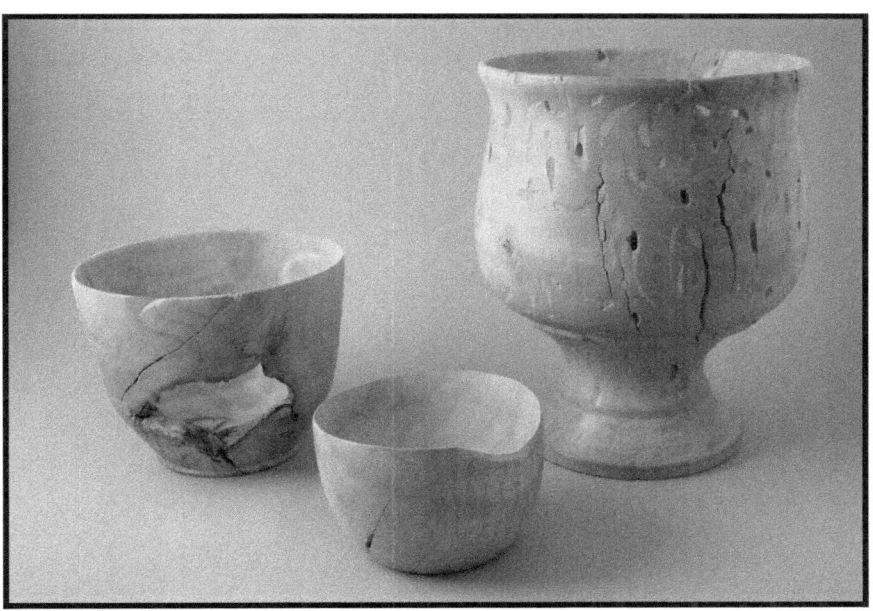

Look at the wooden vessels on the table in front of you. What is the story that their squiggly markings tell? Contemplate:

- What stories do your own scars tell?
- Continue looking at the wooden vessels. Before being fashioned into bowls each was a piece of firewood destined for an ashy outcome. But, something happened! The knotty (naughty?) chunks of fire-fodder were chosen, placed on a turning axis and spun around again and again, encountering sharp tools that pared away bark, grit, and voracious worms.
- Contemplate: How does the Divine intersect with your story to make a new story?
- Prayerfully open your heart and invite the Master Artist to hold you and shape you with a strong, yet delicate touch.
- Lift the vessels to your face and breathe in the fragrance of the potpourri. In that moment, imagine the beauty with which the Divine wants to fill your soul.
- Give thanks, and when you are ready, move to the next station.

Station 3: The Jar of Remembrance

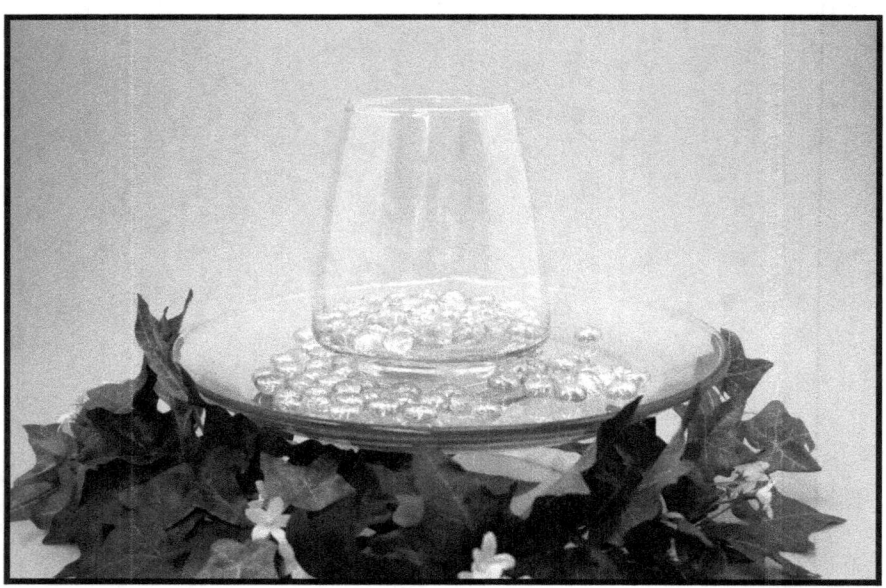

"You have kept record of my days of wandering. You have stored my tears in your bottle and counted each of them" (Psalm 56:8, CEV). These words were recorded long ago by an ancient king as a prayer to his God.

- *Bow your head quietly and allow yourself to feel the Sacred alongside. Visualize the Holy One bowed together with you. Tears stream from loving eyes, falling and mingling with your own, giving assurance that you are cherished and loved.*

- *Prayerfully remember those who have shared your story, those who have shaped who you are, whether for good or ill.*

- *On the table before you is a memorial of remembrance. Help build a memorial to the tears of this world by placing a "teardrop" in the bottle. Then keep one for yourself as a reminder that you are not alone in your journey.*

- *Quietly, prayerfully, give thanks for those whom you love and who love you, and then move to the next station.*

Station 4: The Bowl of Healing Oil

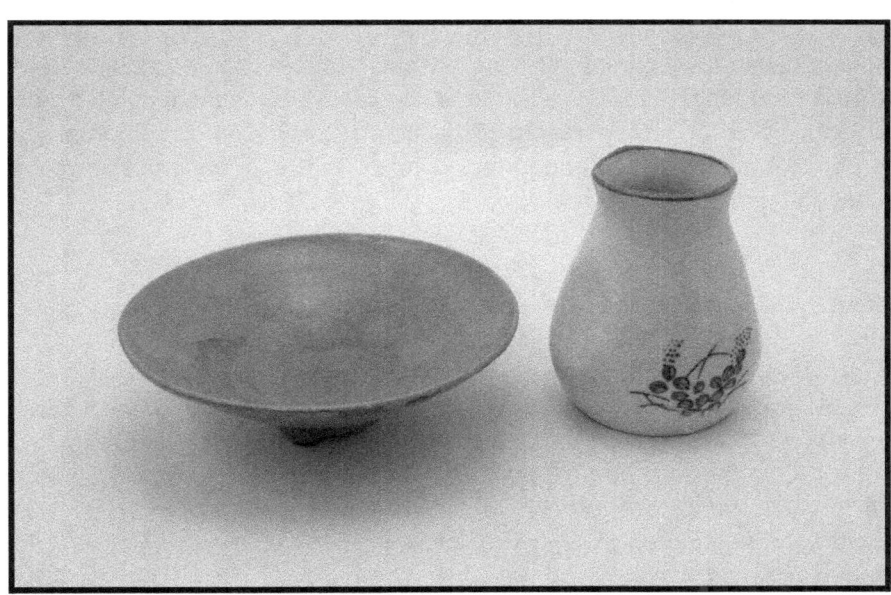

Breathe in the subtle scent of olive oil. It does not overpower, but touches the senses as a gentle presence, bringing a message of selfless caring. Olive oil comes from olives that have been bruised, squeezed, and beaten to bring flavor, light, and life to the world. From ancient times, it has taken on sacred significance, representing the healing influences of both the Divine Spirit and medicinal arts. Thus, to receive an anointing with olive oil is to consecrate oneself to the mystery of the Divine Presence and at the same time affirm the value of human touch.

As an extension of the olive branch, oil placed upon the forehead and hands represents a person's desire to be at peace and to be an emissary of peace. The oil invites the recipient into a prayer for emotional, physical, spiritual, and relational tranquility.

- So, with a prayer of thanksgiving in your heart, dip your finger in the oil.
- Rub the oil on your hands and know that your hands are blessed with all of the love of heaven.
- When you feel ready, return to the world with your hands and hearts anointed for service.

Nurturing Transcendent Values

One day shortly before the Fourth of July, America's Independence Day, I entered our hospital's chapel to regroup after a stressful morning. As I moved around the room, I was disappointed and angered by what I encountered. That night I prayed for an appropriate response, both for myself and for our hospital. In the morning this is what I wrote and sent to all staff:

Feeding Wolves on the Fourth of July

There is a familiar legend passed down from generation to generation. An old man sat with his grandson sharing his life's biggest challenge. "There is," he said, "a fight going on inside me between two wolves. One is evil – hateful, intolerant, and arrogant. The other is good. He is loving, kind, compassionate, humble, and generous in spirit. This same fight is going on inside every other person too, including you." The grandson asked, "Which wolf will win?" The old man replied simply, "The one you feed."

This year as the Fourth of July approaches, my heart is moved to gladness by the freedoms we enjoy, and at the same time, I grieve that a bad wolf so often seems to win against our better nature. For example, not long ago all non-Christian sacred texts selectively disappeared from our hospital's interfaith chapel. Then this month, a prayer rug often used by Muslim co-workers was stolen a third time. After the thefts, only Christian resources remained, making me wonder: what spirit motivates this "sanitizing" of space dedicated for the soul-nurture of all people.

However, rather than attacking and diminishing anyone, I want to feed the good "wolf" that is among and within us all.

As we celebrate America's birthday, I wonder, will our better nature remember what strengthens, sustains, and unites us as a people? The United States Constitution and the Bill of Rights, as I understand them, contain language that is intended to protect minorities from the excessive dominance of a majority culture. Our founding fathers saw rightly that Right is not to be found alone in the majority might of many but in the deeper recesses of the individual human spirit.

In their prescient wisdom they saw that the Right of righteousness appears when each person takes responsibility for the pursuit of his/her own life, liberty and happiness even while seeking to preserve that sacred right for others. This constitutionally mandated respect for minority positions sets American democracy apart from the simple majority-orientation of other democratic systems. (This is also why there is to be no state-church or government-led establishment of religion in America). Thus, as I see it, behaviors such as the removal of non-Christian texts and the repeated theft of prayer rugs from an interfaith sanctum are egregiously disrespectful of the American spirit.

Such behaviors, I believe, are also a repudiation of the truth that paradoxically both transcends and unites people across cultures and belief systems. Please consider the Golden Rule as it appears throughout the world in diverse cultures and religions:

- Native American: "He who does not treat his fellow warriors and squaws and enemies as if they were all good arrows is bound to lose his strings." Black Kettle
- Buddhism: "Treat not others in ways that you yourself would find hurtful." The Buddha, Udana-Varga 5.18
- Christianity: "In everything, do to others as you would have them do to you; for this is the law and the prophets." Jesus, Matthew 7:12
- Islam: "Not one of you truly believes until you wish for others what you wish for yourself." The Prophet Muhammad, Hadith
- Confucianism: "One word which sums up the basis of all good conduct....loving-kindness. Do not do to others what you do not want done to yourself." Confucius, Analects 15.23
- Judaism: "What is hateful to you, do not do to your neighbor. This is the whole Torah; all the rest is commentary. Go and learn it." Hillel, Talmud, Shabbath 31a

When I show disrespect toward the religious beliefs and practices of others, what do my actions show? Is it possible that my behaviors. become "deeds of unfaith" rather than acts of righteousness? How is it for you? Many texts from other cultures and religious traditions might be cited, but perhaps it is sufficient simply to know that within each of us resides a yearning for wellness, including relational well-being. With hope for the Union, may loving-kindness prevail! (See http://www.religioustolerance.org /reciproc.htm for variation of the Golden Rule and related resources).

We replaced our prayer rugs and replenished our interfaith supplies. Months passed, then one day I received an invitation to meet with a grinning group of housekeeping and security personnel. What they shared with me prompted another letter to all staff – this time with joy:

A Season of Stress for Turkeys (And Humans)

One does not need to be a turkey to know that this is a season of exceptional stress. A trip to the chopping block, followed by plucking, stuffing and roasting is not the fate of every bird. Yet, the feeling is all too common. "Swine flu" and a struggling economy, alongside "normal" grief and loss, make this holiday season an occasion of dubious celebration for many people.

Yet, even turkeys have a day of pardon. This is not only a season full of stressors; it is also a time for forgiveness. Earlier this year on the Fourth of July I wrote an article which I shared with our hospital family. In that essay, I wrote about the unauthorized removal of prayer rugs and sacred texts from our hospital chapel, and invited readers to consider how we might live according to "the Golden Rule Across the Religious Spectrum." Black Kettle, a Native American chief said, "He who does not treat his fellow warriors and squaws and enemies as good arrows is bound to lose his strings." It is a good thing when one's arsenal of hope is not broken.

My hopes are very much alive! Last week I was summoned to an unscheduled meeting of hospital security and facilities gurus. Can you imagine my joy to learn that our "wandering" prayer rugs had been found?

It happened this way. Several months ago, apparently some time after the rugs' initial disappearance, after I wrote my Fourth of July letter, one of our facilities workers came across our neatly folded rugs atop a trash bin in our main lobby. He saw that they were "not garbage", but did not then know their origin. Rescuing them, he placed them in his locker for several months, intending to trace their origins later in a free moment. When he finally did so, he learned a little of their history.

Prayer rugs are utilized by persons of faith in various religious traditions (Christian, Muslim, Hindu, etcetera) to create and hold space for communion with the Divine through prayer. They provide a small defined space in the midst of life's chaos to become centered and grounded toward the Holy.

Thus, it is heart-warming to know that The Chapel's prayer rugs have come back home. I believe that the Most Holy One guides the misguided, bringing restoration and forgiveness.

Every year just before Thanksgiving, the White House pardons one turkey in a public display of mercy; but, this pardoning does not stop the presidential family from devouring a different turkey. The Commander-in-Chief's "full and unconditional pardon" is not for all – just for a lucky one. My desire this season – and always – is that love, joy, peace, and the grace of authentic forgiveness and restoration will be experienced by all of us human "turkeys." Now that would be truly scandalous!

Five years have now passed. That season of wolf-like feuding for the soul of our chapel is over, and our chapel remains today a "House of Prayer for All People." The diversely religious and irreligious alike find solace in its space. Now, if only such tolerance could encircle the world!

A Season for Gratitude

My Uncle Pete died just after Thanksgiving when I was a young child. That Christmas my parents, brothers, and sisters and I gathered with my grieving aunt and cousins at Grandpa and Grandma's house.

My beloved Grandpa was out of his preacher's pulpit on the floor with his grandkids, being Santa Claus to them, distributing gifts to each child. As gifts were opened, I noticed that my cousins were collecting a pile of presents that seemed enormous in comparison to my own. It was then that my mother saw something in my eyes and quietly took me to the next room where we talked. It is a conversation I've never forgotten.

"Tommy," she said, "your cousins Ruthie, Ronnie, and Sherry do not have their daddy with them now to give them gifts. So, we spent most of what we had for them. I'm sorry we could not give you more. She then added, "But, Tommy, you still have your Daddy. And isn't he better than a pile of presents?" So very true!

~~~~~~~

While the holidays can be emotionally painful for many, they also bring opportunities to explore and find new coping resources. Walk-through meditations invite people to acknowledge their grief and loss, and simultaneously explore ways toward emotional recovery.

Every walk-though meditation is developed around specific underlying themes. This is especially true around holidays. At such times many feel disconnected from meaning and purpose, from relationships, from hope, and from self-worth. Many struggle to experience forgiveness for known and unknown failures. Thus, our walk-throughs are scripted to address these issues by gently directing thoughts, emotions, and actions toward new possibilities.

The flow from station to station seeks to integrate cognitive, emotional, and behavioral elements, creating a flow from mind to heart to hand. Self-defined changes in thinking, feeling, and doing become a part of how visitors respond. My hope is that each chapel visitor will know, feel, and walk differently afterward. Discovering or reclaiming a sense of purpose, personal value, forgiveness and hope – all these are possibilities as visitors navigate around The Chapel.

WELCOME!

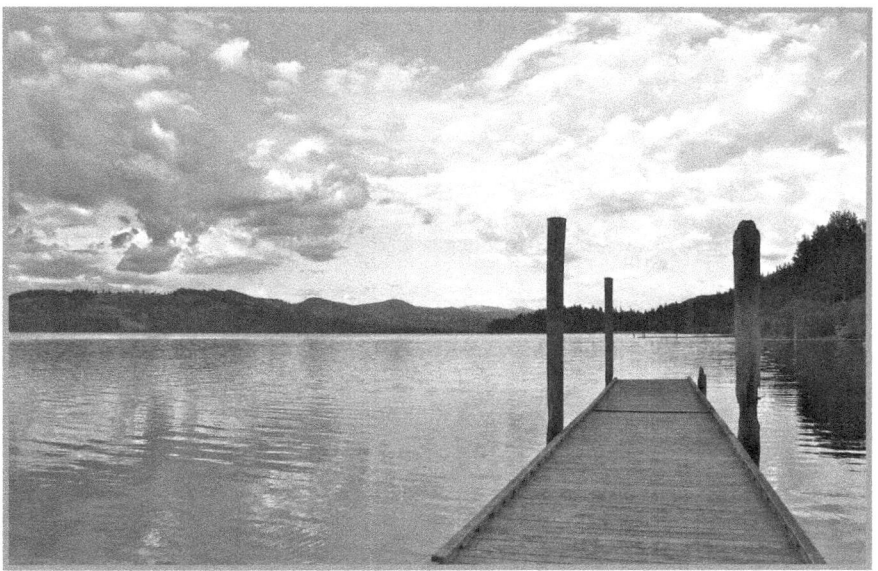

How well are you navigating through the pressures of seasonal activities and continually changing expectations? How about during this holiday season?

Change happens. Chaos is. Yet, beneath the surface of confusion, certain patterns and rhythms are pulsatingly real. For example, consider what happens when you gaze through a kaleidoscope, pointing it toward a light source. The convergence of motion and light causes a chaotic distortion of the horizon though in actuality the horizon remains unchanged. Inside the chaos is a mystery to celebrate.

- As you look through the kaleidoscope of your life, what is on the horizon of your heart? Who and what draws you forward in hopefulness?
- Breathe in and out with deep, cleansing breaths.
- Set aside any pressing concerns.
- Rest and relax.
- When you feel ready, proceed to one of our chapel's resting places. (The stations may be visited in any order.)

Station 1: Give Thanks for Food

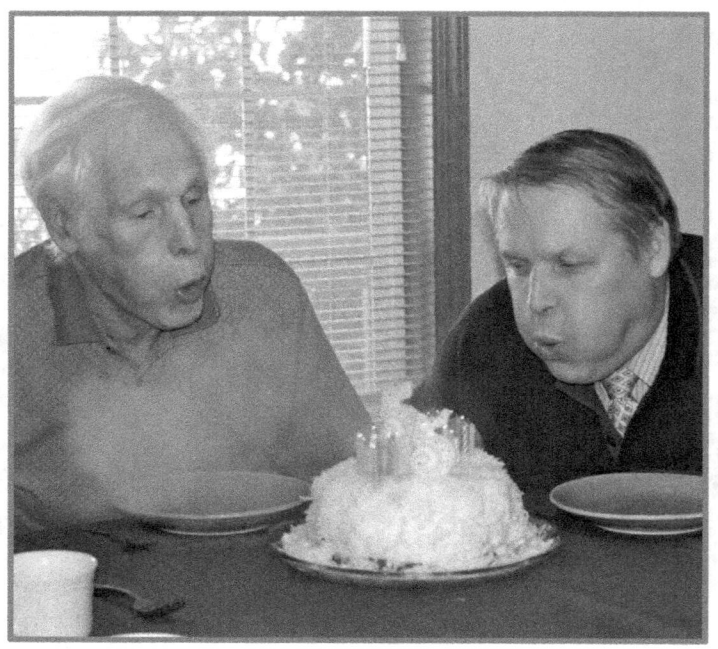

Consider the mysteries of what we eat: *"The harvest is plentiful... first the stalk, then the head, then the full kernel in the head. As soon as the grain is ripe, he puts the sickle to it, because the harvest has come"* (Matthew 9:37; Mark 4:28, 29, NIV). Contemplate:

- *In what ways does the food on your table open your heart to the heart of the Divine?*
- *Contemplate this sacred invitation, "Taste and see that the Lord is good" (Psalm 34:8, HCSB).*
- *Think of your favorite food, and with closed eyes quietly contemplate what it means to invite the Sacred along with that blessing.*
- *When you are ready, proceed to the next station.*

Station 2: Give Thanks for Family and Friends

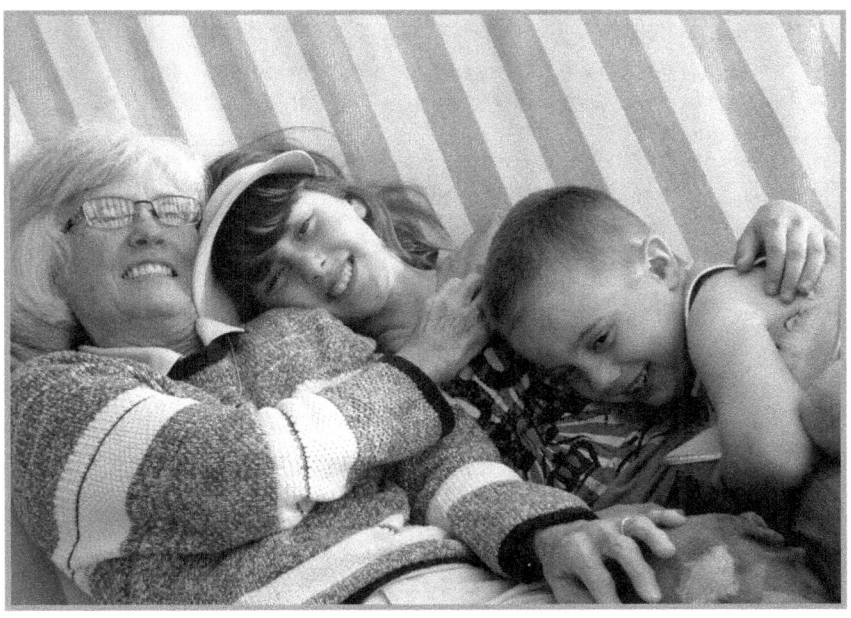

Who can measure the value of caring friends and family? Holidays can hurt or heal. During this season, sit by the fireplace for a while and contemplate how your life is touched by others:

- Who knows you and loves you unconditionally? Are these blood ties or friendship ties? Or, maybe some of both?
- On the card in front of you are some thoughts from Psalm 139 (see next page).
- Reflect on the scriptural passage. Who fits this description in your life?
- What is it like to be fully known yet completely accepted and loved?
- On the table in front of you is also a handout with a "relationship tree" printed on it (see next page). Take one and write on it the names of those persons who make your heart glad. Is the Holy One somewhere there?
- Now, offer up a prayer of gratitude for those who love you and whom you love.
- When you are ready, proceed to the next station.

"LORD, You have searched me and known me. You know when I sit down and when I stand up; you understand my thoughts from far away. You observe my travels and my rest; You are aware of all my ways. Before a word is on my tongue, You know all about it, LORD. You have encircled me; you have placed Your hand on me. This extraordinary knowledge is beyond me. It is lofty!" (Psalm 139:1-8, HCSB).

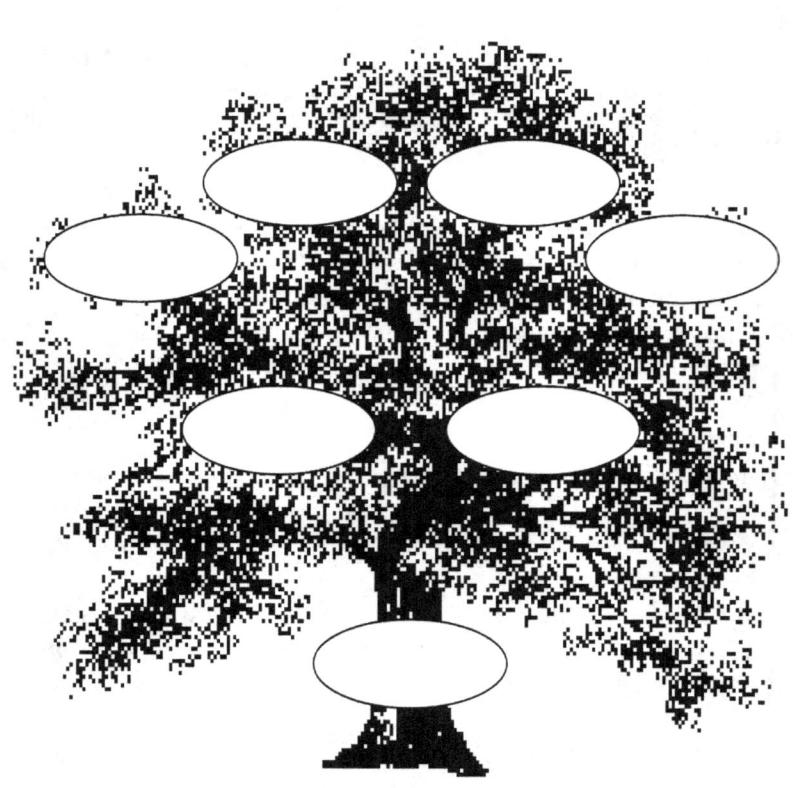

Station 3: Give Thanks for Warmth and Shelter

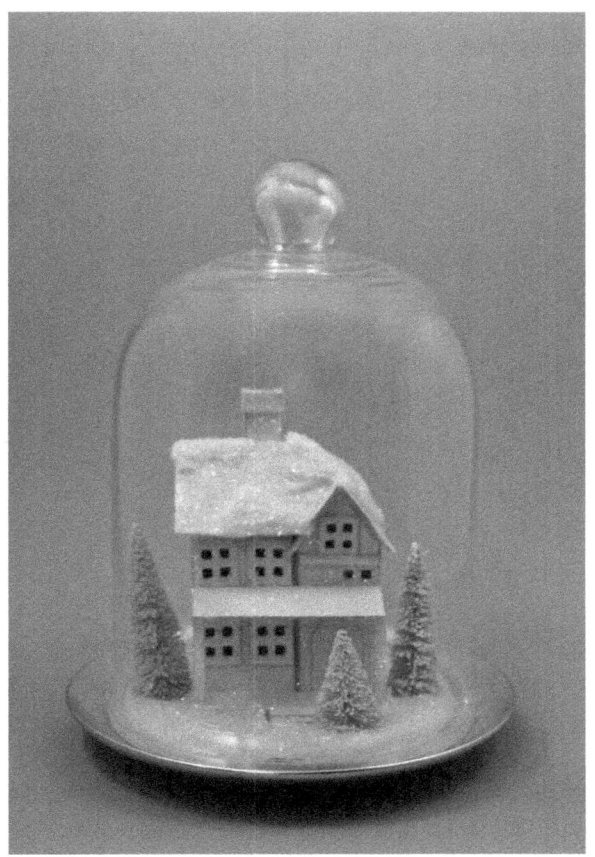

There are many kinds of shelters. For example: different buildings, a tent, a cave, a cardboard box, an umbrella. What makes a shelter a home? What warms the body as well as the heart and soul? Notice the house under protective glass. What might that symbolize to you?

- An ancient king wrote: "Those who live in the shelter of the Most High will rest in the shadow of the Almighty" (Psalm 91:1, NLT). He also prayed: "Let me live in your Holy Tent forever. Let me find safety in the shelter of your wings" (Psalm 61:4, NCV).
- Make yourself comfortable in the chair by the fireplace. Wrap up in the afghan, put your feet up and "sit a spell!" Close your eyes and feel the warmth of heaven's love, surrounding and enfolding you.
- Rest in the shelter of God's care.

Station 4: Give Thanks with Consecrated Hands

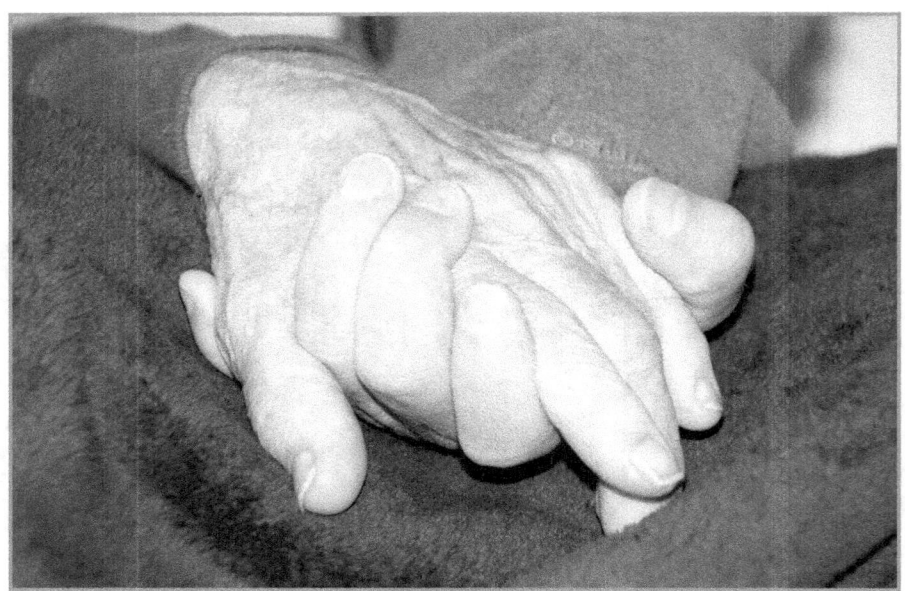

A retired nurse was reflecting on her long years of caregiving. She commented, "I always felt it was so much more than just a paycheck!" How does your own experience with the Sacred translate into how you serve others?

- An apostle of Good News once wrote: "God...will not forget your work and the love you have shown him as you have helped his people and continue to help them" (Hebrews 6:10, NIV).
- On the table before you is a small bowl of consecrated oil. The oil comes to you from olives that have been crushed, squeezed, and drained of their self. It represents a very sacred service to humankind. With a prayer of thanksgiving in your heart, dip your finger in the oil.
- Rub the oil on your hands and know that your hands are blessed with all of the love of heaven.
- When you are ready, return to the world with your hands and hearts anointed for service.

Butterflies and Pieces of Fluff

The transformation of a caterpillar into a butterfly is a powerful metaphor for what happens when institutions redirect energy toward truly *hearing* and responding to the needs, wishes, and choices of patients and their families. Listening is hard work – not unlike the stripping down that a caterpillar does when it emerges from its cocoon.

The transformation of the healthcare experience for patients, their families, and staff is about becoming a community that attends not only to words but to the emotions and spirit of each person. In A.A. Milne's children's classic, Winnie-the-Pooh said, "If the person you are talking to doesn't appear to be listening, be patient. It may be simply that he has a piece of fluff in his ear." While patience toward others is certainly a virtue, digging fluff out of our own ears may be equally or more important. How well do we listen to our core self and that of others?

Chapel retreats are deeply personal fluff-removal adventures. Station scripting invites visitors to listen well to internal voices as they move quietly from station to station.

The Listening Healer

Whether you are a weary skeptic or simply a restless night owl, this is not a journey of hopelessness. It does not matter if you are broken completely or half asleep; you are wholly welcome in this place. This walk-through meditation presents a trajectory of hope and healing. Pause to listen deeply to the Sacred Voice within your soul.

- *Before proceeding to the first meditation station, find a comfortable place to sit or stand for a while.*
- *Breathe in and out with deep, cleansing breaths.*
- *Visualize your stresses floating upward like a butterfly, out of your sight into the heart of the Most Holy.*

On this journey, you will find that each resting place invites communion with silence and with words. In your pausing, listen for the invitation to a rhythmic dance with the Divine Presence. Continue breathing in and out, each time releasing your brokenness and taking in the Spirit of Renewal. With a listening heart, carefully attend to the One who awaits your prayers.

- *Once again, inhale and exhale deeply.*
- *When you feel ready, proceed to the first station.*

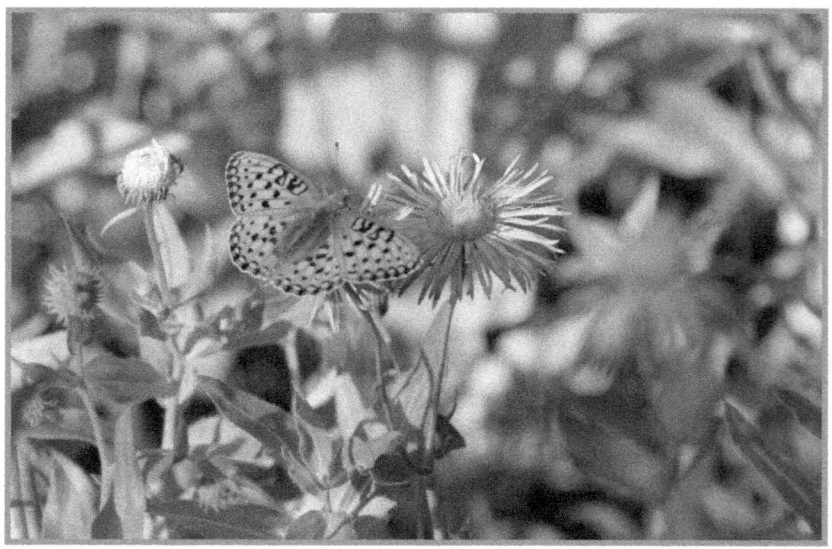

Station 1: The Listening Presence

"For I know the thoughts that I think toward you, says the LORD, thoughts of peace and not of evil, to give you a future and a hope. Then you will call upon Me and go and pray to Me, and I will listen to you" (Jeremiah 29:11, 12, NKJV).

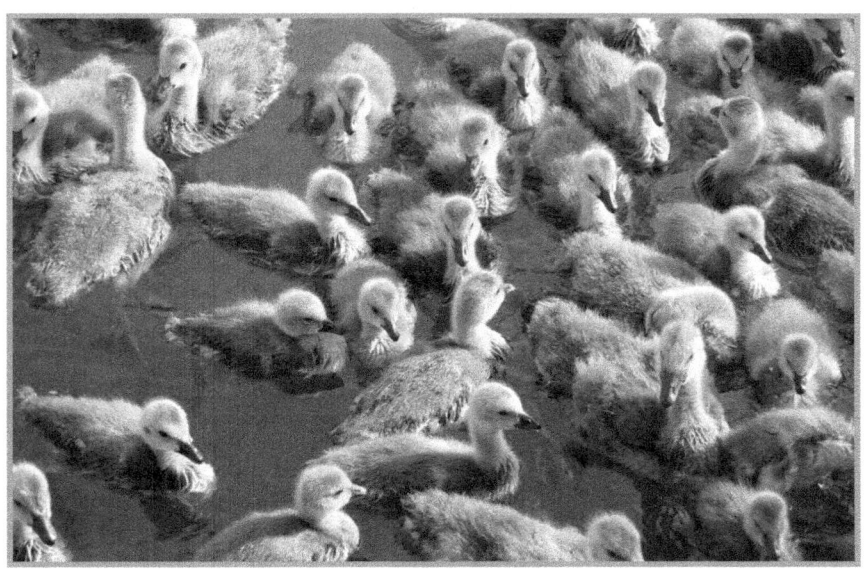

Consider your place among the masses and contemplate all the facets of your life. Ponder places where you've been and where you might go. Identify where you feel the Listening Presence most deeply. Contemplate the paraphrased words of an ancient poet:

"Where can I flee from Your Listening Presence? Where can I go to escape Your Spirit?

"Where can I flee from Your Listening Presence? Lord, you have searched me and known me. If I go up to heaven, You are there; If I make my bed in the grave you are there...

"Even the darkness is not dark to you; the night shines like the day; darkness and light are alike to You, for it was You who created my inward parts; You knit me together in my mother's womb.

159

"I will praise You, because I have been remarkably and wonderfully made" (Psalm 139, NIV).

Prayerfully contemplate: how do you feel when you know that you are fully known AND still perfectly loved by the Author of your life, the Divine Parent who "knit" you together within your mother's womb? When you feel the Sacred moving within yourself proceed to the next station. Visualize yourself being transported to a good resting place.

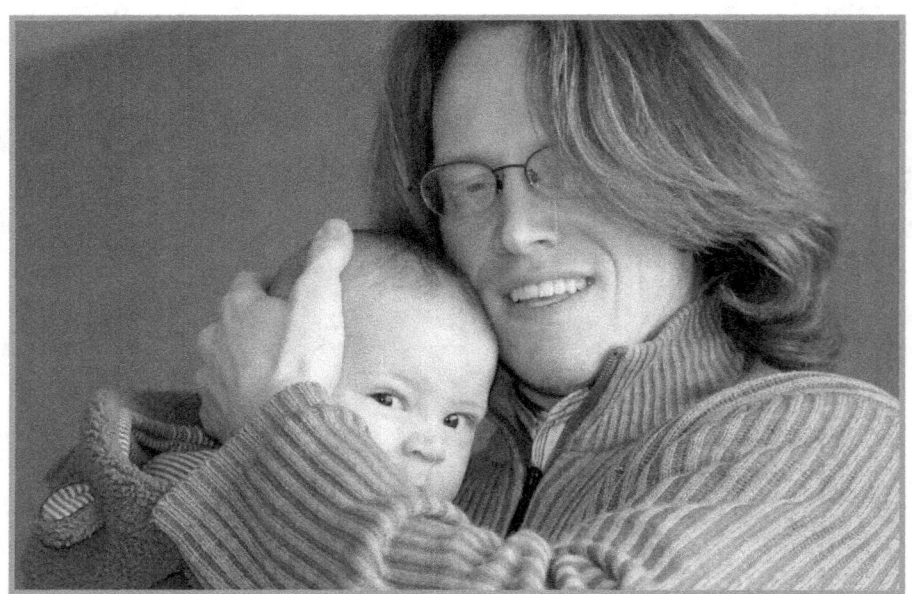

Station 2: Listening, the Gateway to Transformation

The Japanese pictograph for "listen" (聞) is made up of two parts: the character for "ear" (耳) placed within the character for "gate" (門).

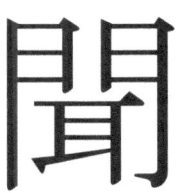

A gate, of course, functions as a point of transition from one kind of experience to another. The presence of a gate also implies a choice: do you pass through or not? How important are ears to you for your choices?

- *Pause to identify times in your life when you stood at a deciding point and needed someone to truly hear and guide you.*
- *Now, imagine yourself sitting within a gate. Where does it take you? Find the entrance to the labyrinth in front of you. As you trace your way toward the center, at each twist and turn, pause to allow the Listening Presence to hear the needs and desires of your heart.*

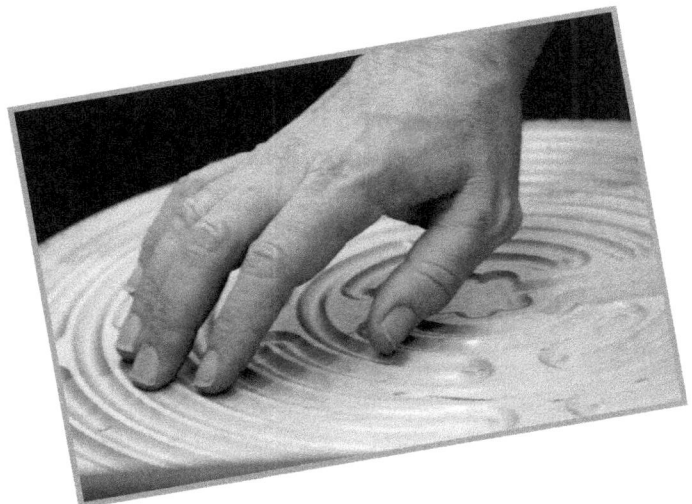

- *Once you've reached the labyrinth's center, stop for a moment. In that space, allow the Divine Spirit to embrace you as you claim the future. With your finger, trace the labyrinth's outward pathway. Pause at each turn to listen heavenward. What might the Sacred be saying to you?*
- *When you are ready, proceed to the next station.*

Station 3: Listening to be a Listener

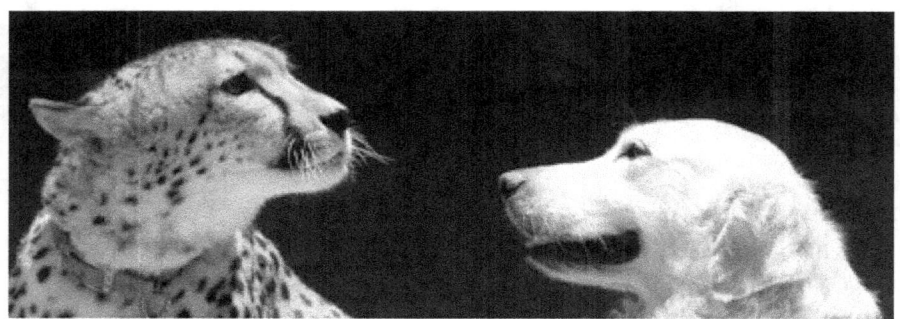

Communication experts say the best listeners are those who know how to listen well to themselves. So, how attentive are you to your inner self? In what ways do your personal beliefs, attitudes, and values help or hinder your capacity to be fully present to others? Contemplate the photograph before you.

- When differences are great, how can you bridge the gap between simple tolerance and friendship? Ponder these words of William Shakespeare:

  Give every man thy ear, but few thy voice;
  Take each man's censure, but reserve thy judgment...
  This above all: to thine own self be true,
  And it must follow, as the night the day,
  Thou canst not then be false to any man.

- If "thine own self" is a true self, what would be the outcome, according to Shakespearian logic? Would your love therefore be more pure?
- Ancient Scripture says that God is always true even though every person be false. His love is therefore also true. What does such love mean to you? How might it transform your inner self and relationships?
- When you are ready, continue on to the next station.

Station 4: Listening with Awakened Ears

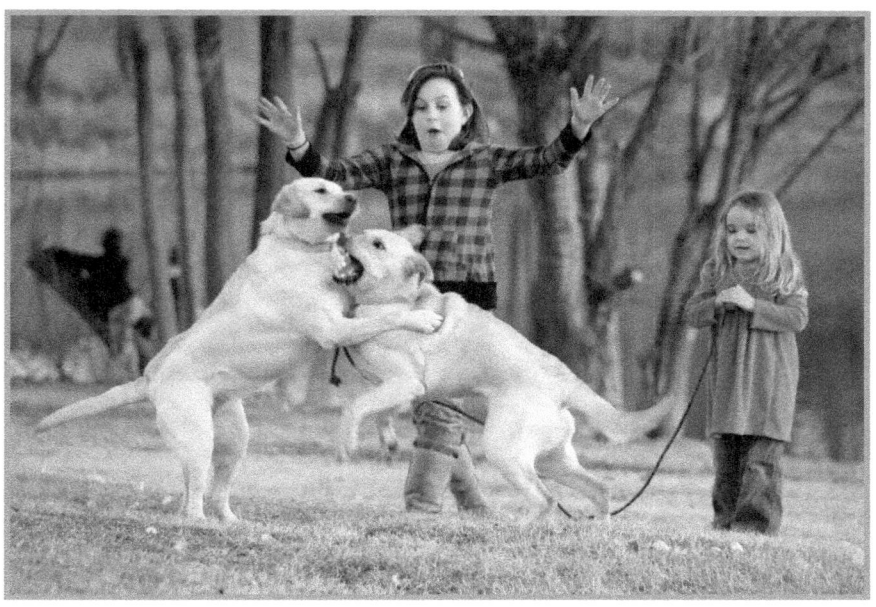

"The LORD God gives me the right words to encourage the weary. Each morning he awakens me eager to learn his teaching." (Isaiah 50:4, CEV).

- What yipping and yapping disrupts your rest? Need help focusing on what's really important?
- Imagine now that you are starting this day all over again. As your senses awaken and light filters through your still-closed eyelids, what are you hearing through the ears of your heart?
- Breathe out your dreams and wishes quietly to the Listening Presence. As you inhale, invite the Sacred Listener to enter all the details of your life.
- Next take a moment to affirm your resolve by partaking of an ancient blessing. On the table in front of you is a small basin of scented oil. Take a drop between your fingers and place it on your right ear. You thereby enter a two-directional covenantal relationship: The Listening Presence pledges to be with you to heal your hearing and to guide you while you vow to attend to the Divine Voice as a servant-learner.

Station 5: Listening in Order to Know

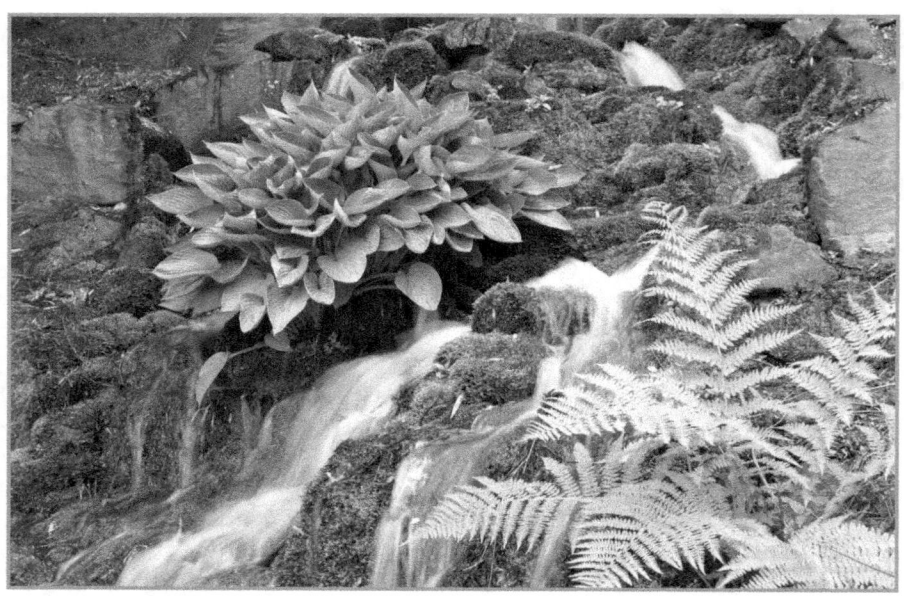

Research indicates that infants first "know" their mother and father by the sound of their voices. Babies will even kick within the womb when Momma sings or Daddy speaks. The Bible says that Abraham, the ancestor of three world religions (Jewish, Christian, Islam), responded with obedience and faith because he "knew" God's voice. Indeed, the Listening Presence is also a guiding presence. How do you recognize the voice of the Sacred in your life?

- Consider these timeless words scribed by one who listened and learned: "Then he led me to the gate...and behold His voice was like the sound of many waters; and the earth shone with His glory" (Ezekiel 43:1, 2, NASB).

- Take time now to allow the sounds of flowing water to cascade over your heart. What does the Voice of Many Waters say to your soul today?

- Listen deeply now to what happened when Ezekiel took time to listen and learn: "The glory of the Lord came into the house by way of the gate...and the Spirit lifted me up and brought me into the inner court; and behold, the glory of the Lord filled the house" (Ezekiel 43: 4, 5, NASB, emphasis supplied).

164

- *Remain where you are until you know that the Listening Presence has heard your heart's yearnings, and affirmed to you that you are not alone.*
- *When you are ready, take one of the cards from the table in front of you and personalize it. Write your name within the blank space. Keep the card as a reminder of how deeply God cares for you.*
- *Go now in the glory of God's peace.*

"For I know the plans I have for you *Tommy* declares the LORD, plans to prosper you and not to harm you, plans to give you hope and a future. Then you will call upon me and come and pray to me, and I will listen to you" (Jeremiah 29:11, 12, *NIV, adapted by T. Becraft*).

EASTER SEASON ENCOURAGEMENT

AN ASH WEDNESDAY INVITATION

How many of us struggle with feelings of personal failure? Wouldn't it be nice if we could live every day with no regrets? How often do we think, "If only I had thought before I spoke" or "If only I had done what I knew I should do"? How often do we struggle internally when we know that we "could've, should've, would've" made a difference for someone else or for ourselves if only we had listened more closely to their heart or our own? Often our best intentions have no more strength than ropes made of confectioner's sugar.

Though broken promises and fractured lives are abundantly common, I have hope. It is a time for renewal. Today is Ash Wednesday, marking the beginning of Lent, a 40-day season of deep reflection and repentance. Long ago Job cried out when he felt the Holy One nearby, "My ears have heard of you but now my eyes have seen you. Therefore I despise myself and repent in dust and ashes" (Job 42: 5, 6 HCSB).

Another ancient seer, Daniel, felt keenly the brokenness of his world and wrote, "I turned to the Lord God and pleaded with him in prayer and petition, in fasting, and in sackcloth and ashes" (Daniel 9:3, NIV).

In that same passage, he records heaven's response. An angel came with an immediate message, "I have come to tell you that you are deeply loved." He reinforced that affirmation by declaring, Help is on the way!

On this day around the world many people choose to receive "the imposition of ashes" upon their forehead. This act memorializes two things: First, it shows that our existence is from "ashes to ashes" except for Divine intervention, and secondly that the Holy One hears the yearning of our hearts and holds us in high esteem, promising grace-filled help for our continued journey unto salvation.

BEYOND EASTER EGGS

"When I was a child, I talked like a child,
I thought like a child, I reasoned like a child.
But when I became an adult,
I set aside childish ways" (I Corinthians13:11, NET).

During this Easter season, do you recall hunting for painted, hidden eggs as a child? What are your memories? For me, egg collecting has few associations with Easter Egg hunts. Instead, memories of egg gathering are linked to memories of my beloved Grandmother. When I was a child, I loved visiting my grandparents' farm where my favorite daily task was helping Grandma collect eggs from the hen house. The chickens cackled and clucked and I loved it. But, even more, it was wonderful to be with Grandma, a very favorite person.

One day when I was just four years old, Grandma sent me outside to play with instructions to not get dirty because she wanted to take me shopping in town later. With her cautions in mind, I therefore wandered aimlessly around the barnyard, solemnly observing Grandpa and Grandma's menagerie. And then with sudden inspiration, I decided to "help" grandma by gathering the eggs for her. Chasing the hens off of their nests, I filled my hands with eggs, and then suddenly realized that I had no egg basket.

But, then, innovative brilliance struck. I carefully placed the eggs in the pockets of my clean bib overalls. I headed back to the house feeling pleased that I could please my Grandma. But, along the way, another brilliant idea struck. I was drawn toward the gaping door of the barn.

Entering, I saw a mountain of hay rising up to the barn's distant ceiling. Yielding to temptation, I turned the mountain of hay into a marvelous playground slide. After several ascents and descents, I descended into worry when suddenly I heard my Grandma calling, telling me that it was time to go to town. In an instant, I realized that all the chicken eggs that I had so carefully collected were well-scrambled and dripping down my legs into my socks and cowboy boots.

But, then, I had one final moment of inspiration. I hid myself in a dark, dark cave in the hay, and waited for light to come. It was there that Grandma found me. I recall my Grandma stripping my sticky, itchy, egg-

smeared bib overalls from me, then hosing me off with cold water while tearfully punishing me for disobeying her request that I not get dirty. But, most of all I remember sitting in clean clothes alongside Grandma later that morning on a park bench, eating Crackerjacks, and basking in the reality of her love.

This month, Christians around the world observe Lent, Passion Week, and Easter. This is a time for remembrance, cleansing, and renewal. It is a time for the scrambled mess of our broken promises to be washed away by heavenly grace. **Chaplain Services therefore invites you to the Chapel for a self-paced, meditation retreat. The Chapel is open 24/7 with Easter-themed meditation stations placed around the periphery of The Chapel.** *You may take as much or as little time as you would like. And in this journey may you find more than scrambled eggs. May you find the Holy One who companions with you on a journey of forgiveness and renewal.*

SKINSHIP FOR ETERNITY – HEAVEN'S EMBRACE

During this season you are invited to journey backward in time to contemplate the life, burial, and resurrection of Jesus Christ. What significance does the past have to you today? Seven stations have been arranged around the periphery of our chapel to help you contemplate and experience that time when Jesus "became flesh and dwelt among us."

Each place invites you to pause, rest and quietly engage in a self-paced journey of remembrance and anticipation. Enter quietly. Resting spots may be visited and experienced in any order. However, if you start at the chapel's garden window and move counter-clockwise, you may find the Lamb of God drawing you progressively closer to a new reality. Release life's burdens as you silently ponder Heaven's gift of infinite love.

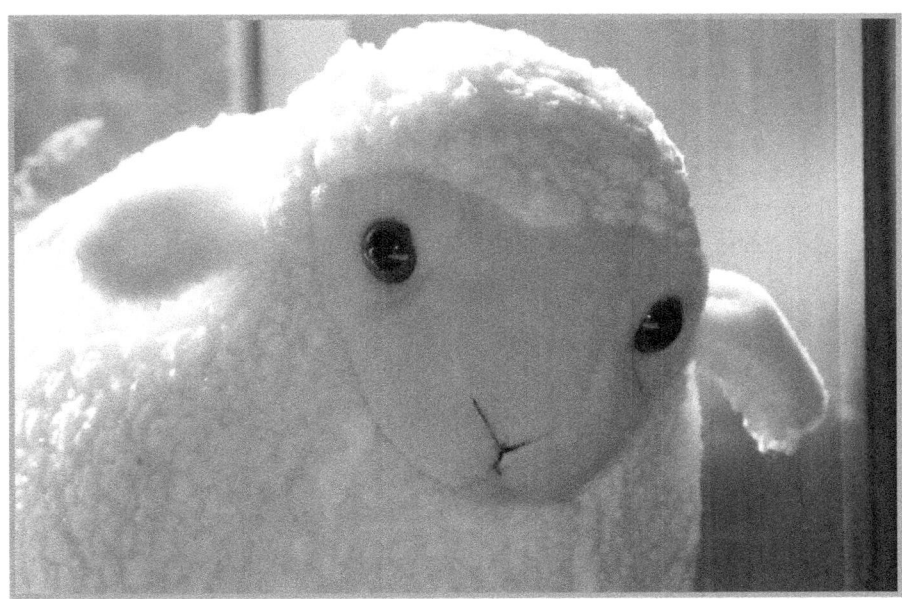

Station 1: Barefoot in the Garden

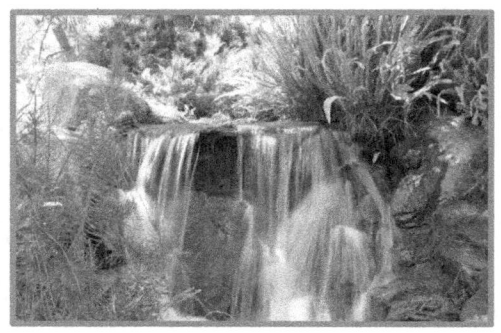

Visualize a special place where pure water flows freely. Sit down and relax. Allow your gaze to fall upon cascading streams of life. Take some deep cleansing breaths. Picture yourself now walking in an ancient garden. An ancient text says of Adam and Eve, "The man and his wife heard the sound of the LORD God as he was walking in the garden in the cool of the day, and they hid from the LORD God among the trees of the garden. But the LORD God called to the man, 'Where are you?'" (Genesis 3:8, 9, NIV). Contemplate:

- *Where are you internally? How are you coping today with personal inadequacies and vulnerabilities? As you watch the flowing water, can you imagine being bathed in forgiveness and re-clothed in hope?*
- *Imagine that you are barefoot and naked, vulnerable before God. Is God doing now for you what He did for Adam and Eve? "The Lord God made garments of skin for Adam and his wife and clothed them" (Genesis 3:21).*
- *Consider: what is the source of this new covering? What does it cost?*
- *On the window ledge in front of you is a fleecy reminder of heaven's gift. Take the lamb in your arms, cradle it, and ask: "how precious am I to Him who has been called 'the Lamb slain from the foundation of the world'"?*
- *When you are ready, proceed to the next station.*

Station 2: Shedding Grief and Pain

"All of us like sheep have gone astray, each has turned to his own way; but the Lord has caused the iniquity of us all to fall on Him. He was oppressed and He was afflicted, yet He did not open His mouth; like a lamb that is led to slaughter, and like a sheep that is silent before its shearers, so he did not open his mouth" (Isaiah 53:6, 7, NASB). Contemplate:

- *How does the ancient past intersect with your experience of life right now? Meditate upon the words above. They were written long ago by the prophet Isaiah as he anticipated the coming of a Savior/Redeemer.*

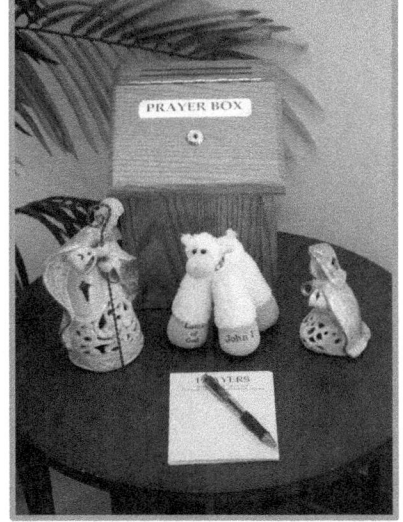

- *The same chapter in Isaiah says, "Surely <u>our</u> griefs He himself bore, and our sorrow He carried." As you examine your heart today, what do these words mean for your past and your future? What happens internally when you embrace heaven's assurance that the Sacrificial Lamb has taken your pain in His own body?*

- *If you are carrying a sorrow of grief deep inside today, please write out the desire of your heart and place it in the prayer box. As you do so, breathe in Heaven's kind assurances of the Savior's presence and exhale the deadening forces of despair. Let your breathing be a prayer of hope.*

- *When you are ready, proceed to the next station.*

Station 3: Shedding Aloneness and Fear

Long ago on a dark night, Jacob, the spiritual ancestor of millions, fled from the murderous anger of his brother Esau after deceiving Esau and their father. The Bible says, "He came to a certain place and spent a night there...and he had a dream, and behold, a ladder was set on the earth with its top reaching to heaven; and behold, the angels of God were ascending and descending on it. And behold, the Lord stood above it and said, 'I am the Lord, the God of your father Abraham and the father of Isaac...and behold, I am with you, and will keep you wherever you go'" (Genesis 28:11-13, NASB).

- With a picture of Jacob's ladder in your mind, consider now the words that Jesus spoke about himself to would-be followers:

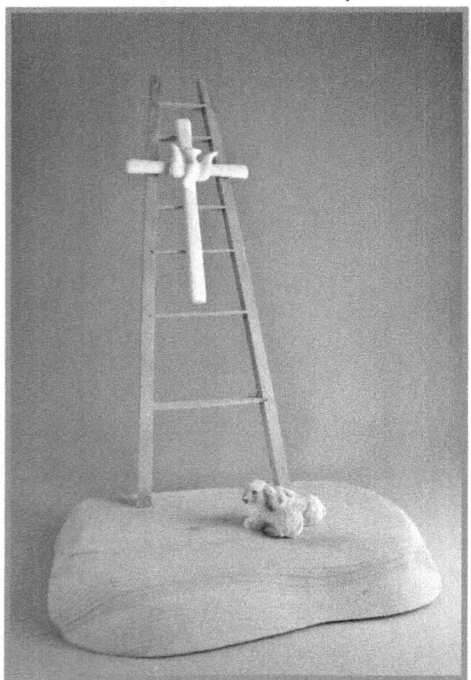

"Truly, truly, I say to you, you shall see the heavens opened, and the angels of God ascending and descending on the Son of Man" (Genesis 28:12, NASB).

- Gaze now at the moving colors on the wall before you. Imagine that you are being carried heavenward on waves of wind and light. Tune your heart to hear the anthem of the ages – "I am with you...you are not alone!"

- As you ascend on the ladder that bridges heaven and earth, what does it mean that Jesus is under your feet? What is in your heart? What is in His?

- When you feel God's Spirit drawing you forward, proceed to the next station.

Station 4: Putting on a Fragrantly Scented Salvation

King David wrote the Shepherd's Song when he was being threatened by some difficult circumstances. Enemies were ready to tear him apart. Read his anthem of hope and ask yourself, "what phrases resonate with my heart?"

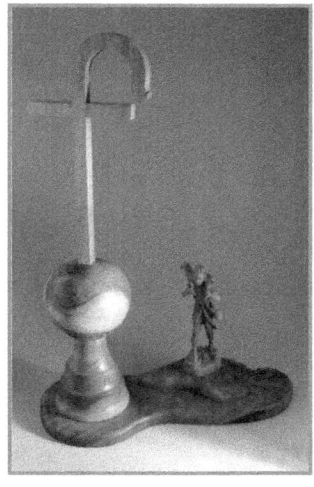

"The LORD is my shepherd; I shall not want. He maketh me to lie down in green pastures: he leadeth me beside the still waters. He restoreth my soul: he leadeth me in the paths of righteousness for his name's sake. Yea, though I walk through the valley of the shadow of death, I will fear no evil: for thou art with me; thy rod and thy staff they comfort me. Thou preparest a table before me in the presence of mine enemies: thou anointest my head with oil; my cup runneth over. Surely goodness and mercy shall follow me all the days of my life, and I will dwell in the house of the LORD for ever" (Psalm 23, KJV). Contemplate:

- When David sang, "my cup runneth over," what do you think he meant?
- What do you need in order to experience a quenching of your own emotional and spiritual thirst? (If you desire to do so, feel free to return to Station 2 to place a request in the prayer box.)
- Observe that the Shepherd anoints your head with oil! In ancient times, fragrant oil was placed upon the head and hands to indicate heaven's consecration of a person both to wellness and royal service. It also represents the soothing kindness of God. Today take a drop of oil from the vessel in front of you and place it on your forehead and hands.
- Pause to savor the sensation of the oil upon your skin and in your nostrils as a pronouncement that you are indeed both known to God and called to be whole.
- When you feel ready, proceed to the next station.

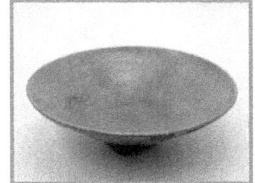

Station 5: Putting on Hope and Joy

Artists of the crucifixion often skillfully drape Jesus' body, compassionately hiding the completeness of His nakedness. Stripped down, flayed, and shamed by those whom he loved, He cried out in the fullness of His human identity, "Father, why...?" What is the impact of this question upon you?

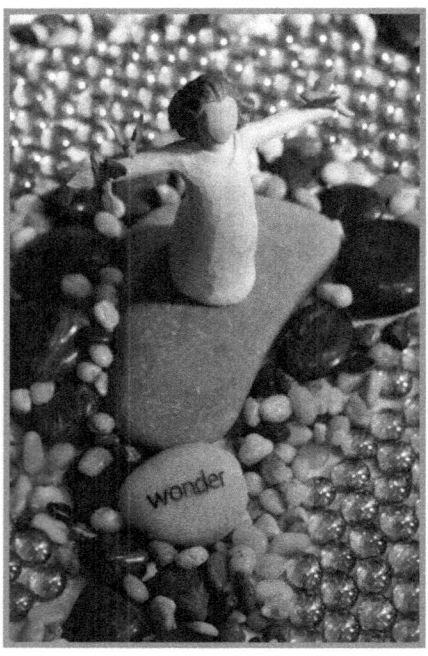

- Ponder now this invitation: "Let us now run with endurance the race that is set before us, fixing our eyes upon Jesus, the author and perfecter of faith, **who for the joy that was set before him** endured the cross, despising the shame, and has sat down at the right hand of the throne of God" (Hebrews 12:3, NASB, emphasis supplied).
- Contemplate: How does "the joy that was set before him" include and touch you? Today are you full of anticipatory joy or grief?
- Consider the sorrow of King David after he committed a terrible deed against another man and the man's wife. When David awakened to know the pain he had caused, he cried out for relief:

"God, create a clean heart for me and renew a steadfast spirit within me. Do not banish me from Your presence or take Your Holy Spirit from me. Restore the joy of Your salvation to me, and give me a willing spirit" (Psalm 51:8).

- The Bible says God forgave David. Contemplate: does Jesus experience joy in forgiving you and filling you with joy?
- When your pain is touched by hope, move to the next station.

Station 6: Putting on the Finishing Touch

On the evening before He died, Jesus ate a festival meal with His closest friends. Included on the menu was the Passover Lamb. On that night, the Bible says, "Jesus knew that the time had come for him to leave this world and go to the Father. Having loved his own...he now showed them _the full extent of his love_" (John 13:3, NLT, footnote translation with emphasis). He then went out from the upstairs room "like a lamb led to the slaughter" (Isaiah 53:7, HCSB).

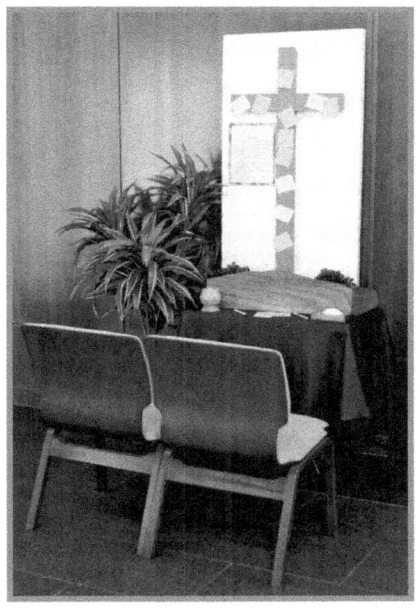

- Contemplate Christ's final hours, focusing on his last words: "It is finished" (John 19:30, HCSB).
- **What is the "it" in your life that you would like to have finished?**
- Before you is a cork-clad cross with some pushpins, pencils and paper. Write down the "it" that you want to be done with and "nail" your paper to the cross. Let God take away whatever you want to give him.
- When you feel unburdened, proceed to the next station.

What is the "it" that Christ is finishing for you today?

Station 7: Putting on Christ's Life

Do you know how much you are loved? "God loved the world in this way: He gave His One and Only Son, so that everyone who believes in Him will not perish but have eternal life" (John 3:16, HCSB). Jesus emptied Himself, descending from heaven's throne to the human tomb. He gave all! But love did not die. The Bible says that early on the first day of the week, after the Sabbath, some of Jesus' followers came to the tomb and found it empty. Contemplate:

- *What does it mean to you today that Christ's tomb is empty?*
- *Imagine that the stone covering the darkness of your soul-tomb has been rolled away. What awaits you now? Hear this promise:*

"No one has ever seen this, and no one has ever heard about it. No one has ever imagined what God has prepared for those who love him" (1 Corinthians 2:9, NCV).

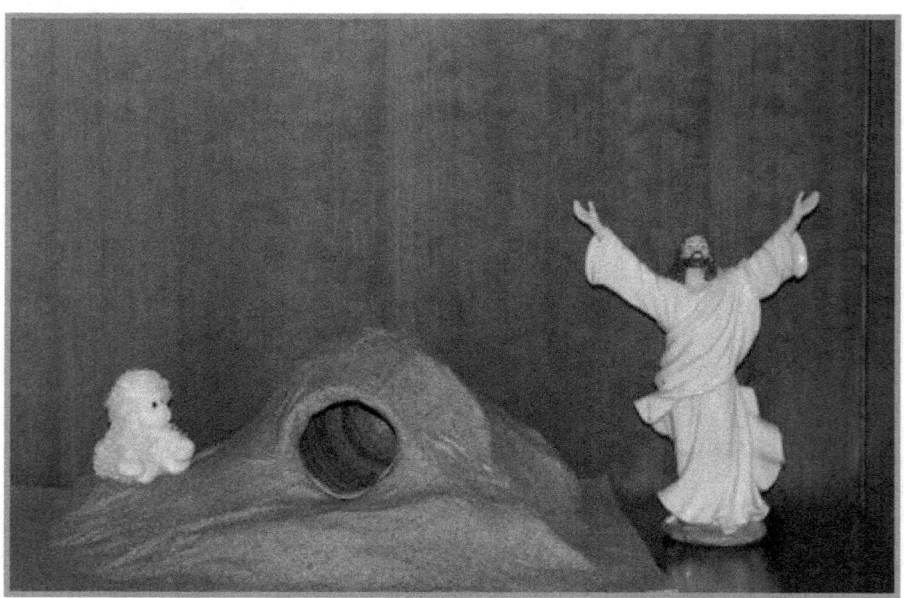

- *Reach now into the tomb in front of you. Fill your hands and hearts with this promise from God: "I will be with you alway, even unto the end of the world" (Matthew 28:20, KJV).*

176

TEARDROPS: TATTOOS UPON THE SOUL

Station 1: What's your story?

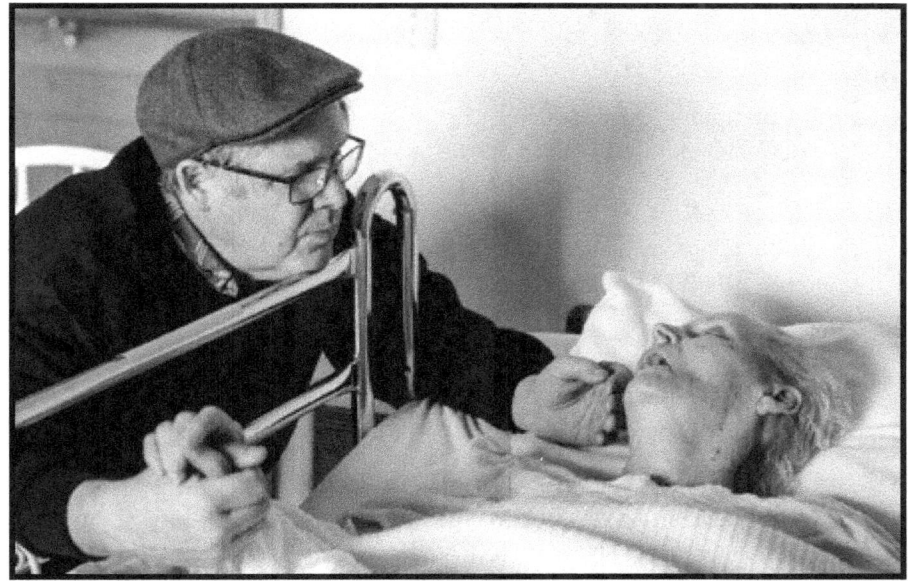

Photo by Tim Becraft

Teardrops are incredibly powerful.
> *They tell a story.*
In the moment that they appear they are real.
> *What do they say?*
Are they tattoos upon the soul?
> *Or are they rainbows in wrinkles*
> > *that last and last as we grow old?*

Contemplate:
- *How do your tears transform you? And what transforms your tears?*
- *Utilize the self-assessment handout (see next page) that is on the table in front of you. Prayerfully identify what brings joy and purpose to your life.*
- *Take time to release your wordless whispers into the Divine Heart.*
- *When you are ready, proceed to the next station.*

A Quality of Life Self-Assessment Tool

Instructions: Circle the number or word that most closely describes your own experience. Then, when you have finished the eight questions here, transfer your scores to the scoring section that follows in order to see your level of vitality.

Healthy Purpose

1. How often do you feel that your life has meaning and purpose?

1	2	3	4	5	6
Rarely	*Seldom*	*Occasionally*	*Sometimes*	*Usually*	*Always*

2. What brings joy and purpose to you?_____
How important is that to you?

1	2	3	4	5	6
Not at all important					*Extremely important*

Healthy Relationships

3. Do you feel closely connected to your family and friends?

1	2	3	4	5	6
Rarely	*Seldom*	*Occasionally*	*Sometimes*	*Usually*	*Always*

4. Who (or what) do you need in order to feel at peace? _____
How important is that to you?

1	2	3	4	5	6
Not at all important					*Extremely important*

Healthy Expectations

5. Do you feel hopeful about your future?

1	2	3	4	5	6
Rarely	*Seldom*	*Occasionally*	*Sometimes*	*Usually*	*Always*

6. Who/what contributes to your emotional and spiritual wellbeing?

_____

How important are those resources to you?

1	2	3	4	5	6
Not at all important					*Extremely important*

Healthy Body

7. Is your physical condition satisfying to you?

1	2	3	4	5	6
Rarely	*Seldom*	*Occasionally*	*Sometimes*	*Usually*	*Always*

8. What energizes and sustains your health? _____
How important is that to you?

1	2	3	4	5	6
Not at all important					*Extremely important*

Now, transfer each of the scores from the Quality of Life Assessment Tool into the corresponding box in this grid. Then total your scores and circle the number at the bottom that most closely corresponds to how you are energized. A higher score indicates greater resiliency and coping resources. A lower score indicates a need to carefully look at how you are responding to the circumstances of your life.

Instructions: Transfer scores from QOL survey into the corresponding boxes below, then place total of scores at bottom.	1 Negative Vitality	2	3	4	5	6 Positive Vitality	
I. **Healthy Purpose** Spiritual Vitality							/6
What brings joy and purpose?							/6
Importance?							
II. **Healthy Relationship** Social Vitality							/6
Who or what is needed in order to be at peace?							
Importance?							
III. **Healthy Expectations** Emotional Vitality							/6
What dreams/goals energize and keep you alive?							/6
Importance?							
IV. **Healthy Body** Physical Vitality							/6
What is essential to sustain your quality of life?							
Importance?							
Total Vitality/Coping Score: **A higher score represents personal clarity, heightened vitality and a greater capacity to cope with life's uncertainties**							/48

Negative Vitality		Moderate		Positive Vitality
0	12	24	36	48

If you could awaken tomorrow to a perfect world,
what would that look like?
What would it feel like?
What hope do you have for transformation?

179

Station 2: What moves your heart?

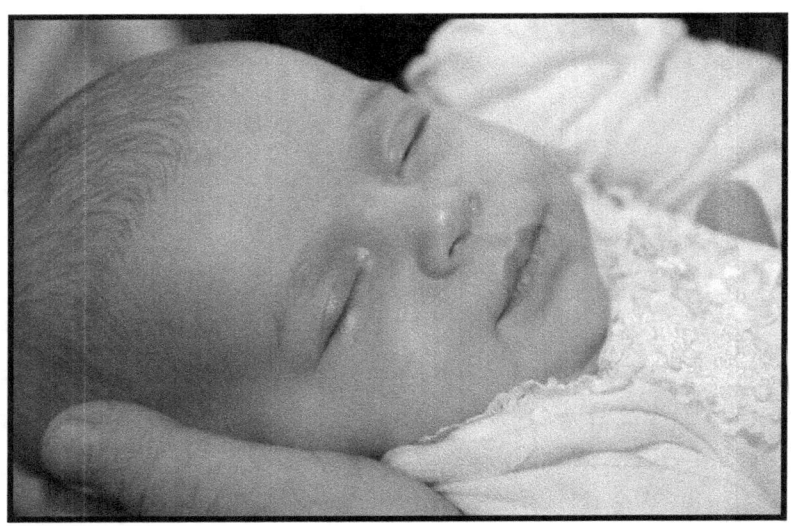

Can you name the feeling that comes to you when you see a sunrise or sunset, or hear the spontaneous sounds of innocence? Consider: When was the last time you paused to feel the touch of the Sacred upon your skin, upon your eyes, upon your ears, upon your soul? Have you experienced Holy Spit?

> *HOLY SPIT*
> *Tears are a mother's spit applied upon a dirty face.*
> *Weeping is her hand firmly gripping the ear*
>   *of a thoughtless rascal*
>   *who has forgotten where he's bound.*
> *Tears are the caress of a grace-filled parent.*

Long ago, Isaiah, a weary sage, sang out to God, "You chose me to know you, to believe in you, and to understand... Nothing can snatch me out of your hand" (paraphrase of Isaiah 43:11-14).

Imagine yourself gripped in gentle, healing, cleansing hands. In those hands, what does God want you to experience in the Holy Presence?

When you feel confident that you are held securely in Cleansing Grace, proceed to the next station.

Station 3: Is life's garbage overwhelming you?

Behind my home is a sawdust sanctuary full of tools and projects. I retreat there to hammer, saw, drill, plane, chisel, sand, or simply ponder. Sometimes an accumulation of broken tools and unusable scraps muddles my pondering and projects. So, I periodically take inventory. Broken or unusable items are moved into a pile that I may look at and ponder for a while before hauling them away. In the same way, prayerful soul-searching tells when it is time for a trip to unload at the Garbage Transfer Center.

For many of us, unloading what no longer works may be painful, but it creates space and opportunity for more productive pondering and creativity. This might mean giving up dysfunctional beliefs and practices. Yet it opens the way for heaven's pure breath to enter and ride the highways of our being.

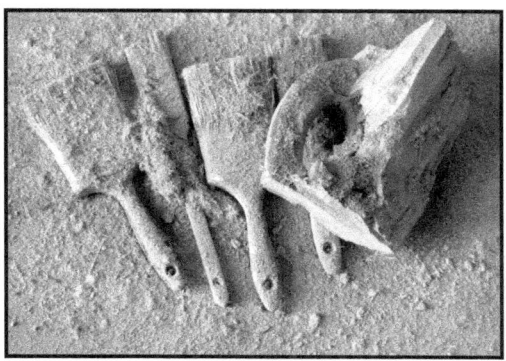

Ponder for a while:
- What is the debris in your life that you want to discard?
- What will replace what no longer works for you?

SAWDUST
Tears are the soul's response to sawdust
  Welling up to cleanse the vision.
Weeping is the squeegee wiping across the heart,
  Removing the debris and crud of our craftsmanship.

- Utilize this time and this place to assess and unload the internal garbage that is getting in the way of your wellbeing.
- When your heart feels lighter, proceed to the next station.

Station 4: What is your legacy?

There is a song, "My Time on Earth," popularized by a then-young singer, Billy Gilman. It says:

> *"It is not the length of life or the depth of the grave.*
> *In the end, we'll be measured by the love that we gave."*

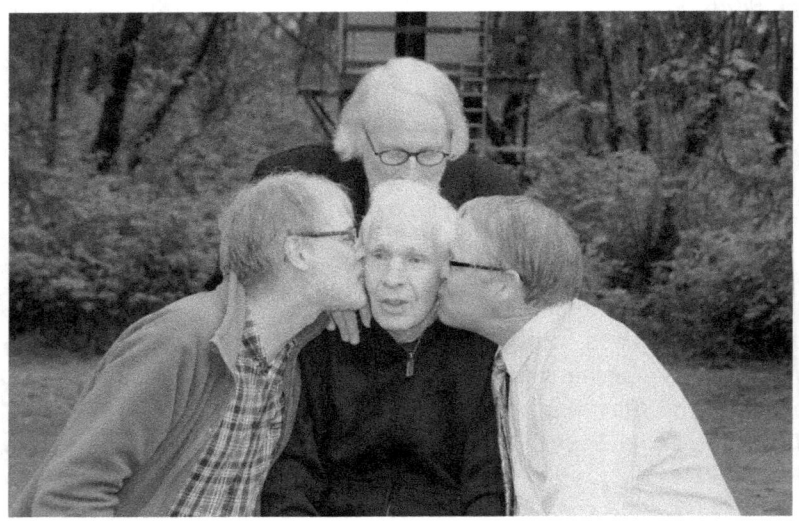

Contemplate: How have you showed love toward others? Do you feel inadequate, or that you've failed? Do you want one more chance?

> *NON-VERBAL PLEAS*
> *Tears are silent screams, unmouthed prayers,*
> *Falling into God's jar-heart.*
> *Weeping is spilling self*
> *Into Sovereign hands.*
> *Tears are letting go,*
> *Trusting to Heaven's tender care,*
> *Resting, cherished, cleansed.*

- *Consider this promise: "Even to your old age and gray hairs I am he, I am he who will sustain you. I have made you and I will carry you" (Isaiah 46:3, 4, NIV).*
- *Pause and invite the Lord to pick you up and carry you to the next station and beyond.*

Station 5: Is life out of control?

Thoughts and feelings don't ask permission. Neither do tears. Sometimes they are chemically triggered by chemotherapy or through neurological damage after a life-altering stroke. Is there hope in the face of the uncontrollable?

Contemplate the cycles of life: Life pushes up from the ground, blossoming, and then falls as flower petals on the sod in winter. What 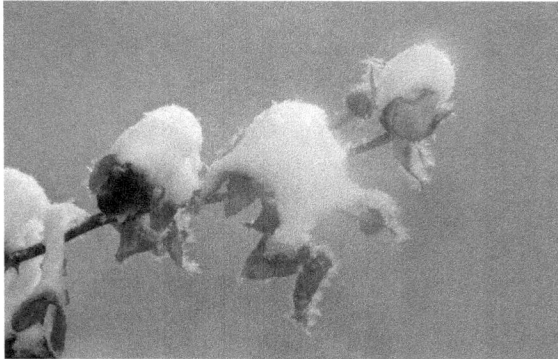 *then? Water lifts in clouds and drifts over land, falling in snow, sleet, hail, rain, and dew drops. What then?*

Are tears really passively compliant with facial terrain, or do they transform the face down to the level of the heart? What trickles deep within you? What rises from within?

ICE SHARDS
Tears are the tip of a melting iceberg,
       Casting shards of brokenness into the deep.
Weeping is the crumbling of fragile foundations,
       Dropping the heart into darkness to reemerge in rainbows.
Tears are droplets of dreams, the splash that mist,
       Arising in light to bathe the soul.

Someone well acquainted with personal and societal woes described to God the light that came to him after tears:

"You have turned my mourning into joyful dancing; You have taken away my clothes of mourning and clothed me with joy, that I might sing praises to you and not be silent. O Lord my God, I will give you thanks forever" (Isaiah 30:11, 12, NLT).

When you feel your heart start to dance again, move to the next station.

Station 6: Have you heard heaven's pledge to you?

The Author and Editor of Life stretches out gentle hands to touch the parchment of our hearts, pledging allegiance to our wellbeing. We feel the imprint of the divine pen, reforming our past, scripting us with hope. Forgiven and revived, we are assured that a better day is coming.

INK DROPS
Tears are drizzle drops of the Infinite,
    Spilling from Heaven's soul-portal.
Weeping is the quill in the hand of heaven's aspiration,
    Opening the soul to inspiration.
Tears are ink on parchment,
    Bringing to fruition the sacred story.

The Author of Wellness will write a new ending.
    Grief, crying and pain will fly to oblivion.
"Passing away" will pass away.

NO MORE RUSTING, ROTTING, OR EMPTY CHAIRS!

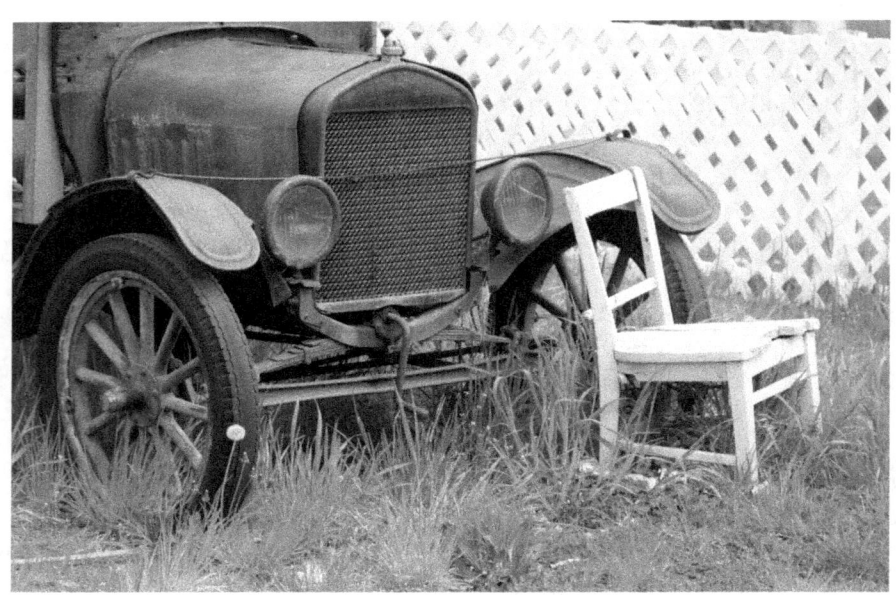

CREATING PAUSING PLACES

For family members of a hospitalized patient, bedside vigils are a lot like a merry-go-round, but without all the merriment. There is an endless up-and-down, around-and-around parade of doctors, nurses and other visitors, each dancing to the bells and whistles of constantly changing rhythms. If one blinks for an instant, one might miss something important. Thus, family members often feel compelled to stay close by their loved one, studying the rain of fluids from IV bags, monitoring the approach of thunder and lightning on bedside screens, and anxiously awaiting news that the storm threat is moving past.

At such times, it is hard for caregivers to leave the bedside and seek solace and strength in The Chapel. The Chapel feels distant and inaccessible, even while prayer is claimed by them as an important coping resource. Because of this, and because few hospitals are staffed with enough chaplains to go wherever prayer is desired, it is important to find other means to make spiritual care available.

One way to do this is by creating "chapel extensions" throughout the hospital. At Kadlec every unit, every floor, every corridor now has a pausing place that invites passersby to stop for a moment to reconnect with hope. No one has to travel far or spend much time away from their loved one in order to renew emotional and spiritual strength in a place of prayer.

We call each of these chapel extensions "The Pausing Place." Each is equipped with four elements:
- An invitation to pause
- A finger labyrinth
- A prayer box
- Printed resources

Since establishing these unit-based pausing places prayer requests have multiplied over 10 times.

The invitation is laser-engraved, framed and mounted on the wall. Here is what it says:

The Pausing Place

Never is a prayer lifted heavenward without the Holy One reaching out in compassion to touch the wounded spirit of the broken-hearted.

Even before we articulate the yearnings of our hearts, heavenly grace descends, nudging us toward healing. As our hearts and hands open toward heaven, the mighty arms of the Most Holy One reach out to enfold us, bringing us rest and peace. In those faithful hands is wellness.

The Labyrinth and the Prayer Box

So, pause in this place and let your hands grasp hope. In front of you is a wooden labyrinth. Put your finger at the labyrinth's entrance and then slowly trace the pathway toward the center. At each twist and turn, breathe out the desires of your heart. When you arrive in the middle, linger for a moment to prayerfully release your anxieties into the heart of the Sacred One.

Next, slowly move your finger back to where you started. Take time to say good-bye to despair and to embrace the assurance that you are not alone in life's journey.

Now, pause a little longer and place your prayer requests and expressions of gratitude in the prayer box. Kadlec's spiritual care team checks this box regularly and is committed to holding you in prayer.

THE FINGER LABYRINTH

The labyrinth is an ancient tool used across the spectrum of cultures and religious traditions to help persons slow down long enough to anchor themselves to whomever and whatever relieves inner tension. It is a neutral device that does not prescribe what to believe, think, or feel. It simply provides space, time, and opportunity for persons to look inward, outward, and upward in their quest for a more balanced and well-integrated life.

THE PRAYER BOX

Each prayer box was made to match the décor and space limitations of the hospital unit for which it was destined. Those placed in corridors have a wall-hugging profile so that they do not interfere with passage of hospital gurneys and other equipment. Some are four-legged, waist-high, free-standing receptacles placed in waiting rooms. Those in consultation rooms are appropriately compact and placed on side tables. Wherever placed or however designed, each box reminds that the journey to wellness is traveled in community with others, both human and heavenly.

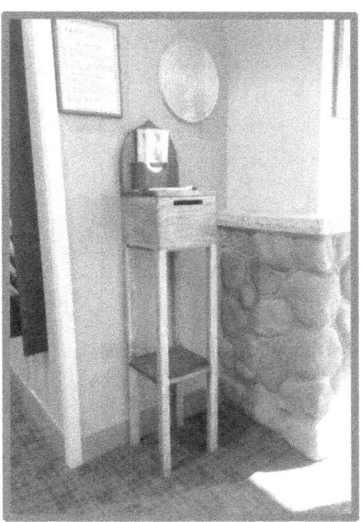

PAUSING PLACE PUBLICATIONS

Two or three printed resources, no more, are placed alongside each prayer box. (We don't want to overwhelm the overwhelmed!)

- *Prayers for the Sick and Tired* is a hospital-published collection of prayers from diverse cultures and religions. While the booklet provides words of transcendent worth, it also educates regarding religious and cultural tolerance.

- *Emotional and Spiritual Care When the Body Breaks: Chaplains, Consultants for Wellness*. This is a tri-fold brochure introducing Pastoral Care Services.
- *Crossing the Bridge: A Guide for End of Life Issues* is a hospital-published 48 page booklet with practical information for patients and family members who are facing life's most difficult choices. (This booklet won the 2011 Planetree Award for Spirituality and Diversity.) Updated regularly, it is used extensively with families by hospital staff as part of conversations before, during and after a death has occurred.

STUFFING THE CROSS
AND EMPTYING THE WINEGLASS

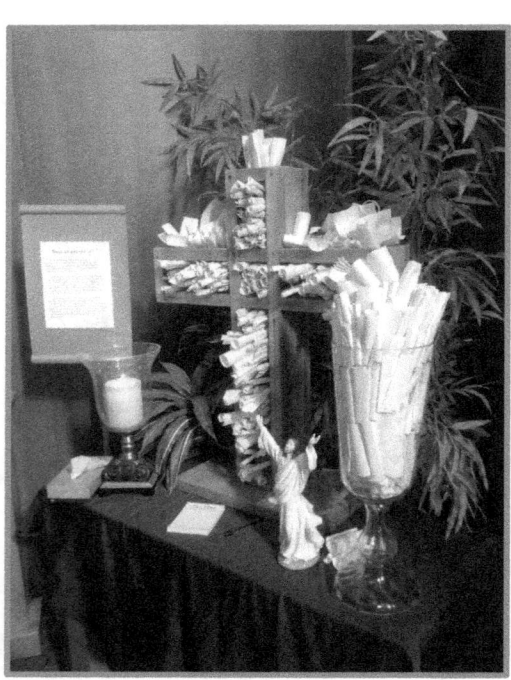

Though there are prayer receptacles throughout the hospital, none has drawn more visitors and generated more outpouring of pain and hope than a hollow, stone-filled cross situated in the corner of The Chapel. The cross's walls are made with wire mesh and the interior is filled with river rocks. Visitors write their requests on paper and insert them into the cross's many openings, sliding them between stones. Over time every nook and cranny becomes stuffed with petitions.

Like life, The Chapel's cross is not tidy, pretty, or smooth. Its contents threaten to fall out like tear drops. Each day new prayer notes fill vacant spaces and in so doing they press against other petitions creating a scene that is paradoxically both ugly and beautiful. It forms a picture of sacred community holding one another together in rocky, rough circumstances.

In order to provide space for new prayer requests, chaplains periodically transfer older requests to a large adjacent glass jar that is shaped like a wineglass. Each request is handled respectfully and held in trust for a special time of release.

On spiritually significant days such as Ash Wednesday, the "wine glass" is poured out, and all accumulated requests are burned in a ritual of relinquishment in the hospital's healing garden. Smoke rises up like incense ascending forever into the Heart of the Holy. In this way, chaplains continually open and hold space for the outpouring of pain, grief, and hope.

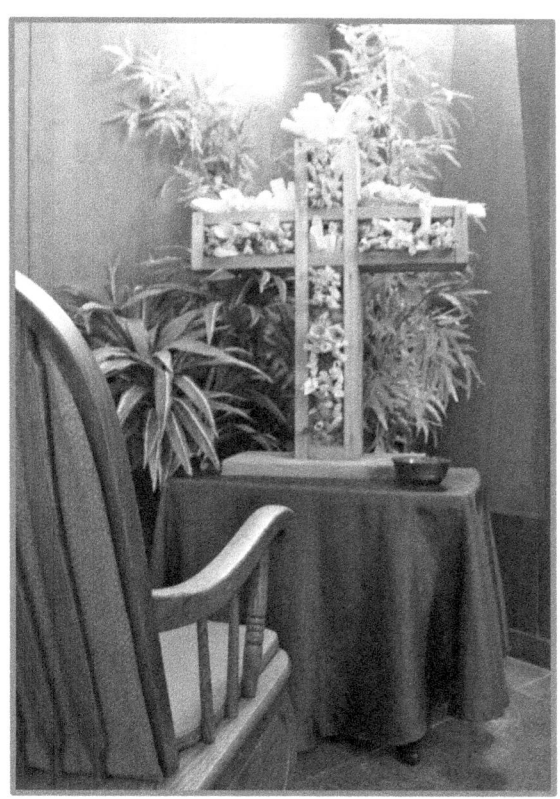

*Earthly friends
may lose their ability
to help us, however much they
desire so to do; but He remains
throughout eternity the
infinitely Rich One.*

George Mueller, *Answers To Prayer*

Chapter 5

FAVOR
THAT LASTS FOREVER

How long does it take to discover the fickleness of friendships? I was barely 10 when I excitedly packed my sleeping bag, flashlight and other essentials for an overnight hike up Mount Bally. It was one of those warm early summer nights when the moon's crescent cast quirky shadows through ghostly evergreens onto the winding logging road that ascended toward the snow-capped summit. Nothing could be more fun than this, I thought, as I kicked pinecones through the dust. Adult leaders of our troop, marched us forward, chanting, "Left, right, left, right...I left my wife at home with seventeen kids." It was great to be with friends. Certainly I did not want to be left behind.

Midnight came and went, and at last we arrived in a sloping clearing where we rolled out our sleeping bags under a star-filled sky. The sounds of coyotes echoed through nearby gullies. Stories of bears, mountain lions, and other ravenous critters flowed freely from the lips of our fearless counselors. It was a night for my active imagination. Who knew what might be lurking in the shadows nearby? I truly did not want to be left behind. But, I was.

Rising early before daybreak, my friends and I pushed toward the summit. We were greeted by a ball of fire on the eastern horizon. It touched my soul with something profoundly mysterious. I took off my summer jacket and spread it beneath me on the snow pack and sat down. I felt this deep fullness in my spirit, yearning to soak in the beauty. I saw a distant river glistening like a golden ribbon winding through my hometown.

I stretched out upon my back and watched strands of silky clouds stretch into the distance overhead. Throughout the past year I had spent significant time with my grandfather whose love for God's creation was evident in his capacity to identify flowers, birds, fungi, bugs, and mammals (even by their Latin names) and tell stories about them. My memories took me into a dream-like reverie. It was as if I was standing on the threshold of something important. Grandpa often spoke of God as a personal friend who hears the desires of our hearts. How could I, I wondered, understand the vastness of God's love, power, and presence?

Then the coolness of the snow began to penetrate through my jacket to my skin. I awakened and looked around. The desolate snowfield stretched out before me. Gone were all of my friends. Gone were my troop leaders. Gone was my strong sense of the Divine. I was alone, left behind. In my panic, I raced around the crusty snowcapped field trying to see what direction my companions had gone. I yelled. I shouted. Tracks led many directions. I was lost. Abandoned. Scared. Which trail to take? Nighttime ghosts lurked in every direction. I wept, and prayed, and blubbered, and started walking down a road that seemed somewhat familiar.

Ten minutes, a half hour, forty-five minutes, an hour! It seemed like forever before I heard noises coming up the trail toward me. The troop converged on me like vultures on a dead opossum, yelling, "What happened? Where were you?" Before I could answer, "Up there!," my closest friend, Cecil, saw my face and burst out laughing and taunting, "You've been crying! Cry baby! You're a cry baby!" Others joined in. I felt keenly the fickleness of friendships!

Not only did I feel betrayed by Cecil and the pack mentality, I felt abandoned by myself. I could not control my feelings of outrage and injustice. I lost further control of my tear glands, thereby escalating the cycle of taunting.

In adulthood, it is yet easy to be caught in an emotional cycle that can spiral out of control. For me, the only way to break the cycle of emotional volatility is to put a "stick" in it – a giant beam. When I turn to the cross of Jesus, my mind and my emotions shift away from self-absorption in recognition that I have a Lord who died and rose again as my everlasting friend. I am not alone no matter the circumstances of life.

Fall came to Sapporo on the far northern island of Japan, and I needed a break from the relentless grind of people's expectations. So, I headed for Mount Maru, leaving the bustling city behind. Language school was now in my past, and I was interning under a veteran Japanese pastor, learning from him what I had not learned in ministerial training classes back home in America. "I work every day and haven't taken a day off in ten years," he proudly told me. Not exactly the lesson I had wanted to learn! His work ethic exceeded my capacity to comprehend or easily accept. How could I find time for family if I was expected to match his pace from morning to night, day after day, year after year? Body, mind and spirit rebelled. How could I manage all my responsibilities?

Sweat broke out on my forehead matching the anxieties in my heart as I ascended the trail. Each step over and around rocks and roots carried me through shadows. Blue sky and sunshine penetrated in patchwork patterns on needles and nettles. Scriptures danced in my head. "I lift up my eyes to the mountains - where does my help come from? My help comes from the Lord, the Maker of heaven and earth...He will not let your foot slip...The Lord watches over you."

Breaking out of the trees, the path meandered to an overlook of the valley below. In that spot, I happened upon a lichen-covered stone with ancient pictographs etched into its surface: 山の神 – *yama no kami*, God of the Mountain. There in that place, a song cycled through my head. It was a song that I first heard on a Sabbath evening after an intense week of language learning just a year earlier. I had become discouraged by my slow progress and was wondering if I would ever be able to approximate the Japanese verbal skills of my two-year old child.

On that night, while my son Andy clambered back and forth over me as I lay on our living room floor, his mother sat at the piano nearby and sang, "When I'm low in spirit I cry, 'Lord, lift me up, I want to go higher with Thee.' But, the Lord knows I can't live on the mountain, so He picked out a valley for me. He leads me beside still waters, somewhere in the valley below; He draws me aside to be tested and tried, but in the valley He restoreth my soul" ("In the Valley He Restoreth My Soul," Hymn No. 19, *Country and Western Hymnal*, Singspiration, Division of the Zondervan Corporation).

When pressed from every side, King David cried out "Where does my help come from?" God gives a timely answer. The Creator is not only on the mountaintops, but is also Companion everywhere. The modern counterpart to David's lament proclaims, "It's dark as a dungeon and the sun seldom shines, and I question, 'Lord, why must this be?' But He tells me there's strength in my sorrow, and there's victory in trials for me...In the valley He restoreth my soul."

Standing beside the ancient monument, I remembered that night of singing and was strengthened. From the lichen-encrusted monument atop Mount Maru, I returned to the valley with an awareness that rivers flow through. The high places of the earth are no more the dwelling place of the Sacred than are the low places. In fact, God reigns over all.

Anticipating Joy

The darkest places in life are often where the Holy works most mightily. Bamboo farmers know that when a seed is planted beneath the soil, a harvest like no other will eventually emerge and suddenly change their family's fortunes. Yet, the blessings do not come suddenly.

The first year, the farmer plants, waters, fertilizes, and waits.

The second year, he waters, fertilizes, and waits. Nothing. Out of sight roots creep, but above ground, there's not a sprig or a peep.

The third year, there is not a hint of green. He is gentle with his spade work. The work of life in darkness must not be disturbed. He waters, fertilizes, and trusts.

The fourth year, he waters still more, piling on hope.

In the fifth year, the seed's creeping becomes peeping and finally there is leaping. In 90 days, a tiny nub thrusts itself 60 feet into the air, strongly held by a root system that can endure the divisive forces of an earthquake. A sanctuary for life has been formed in darkness.

To survive and thrive as a caregiver requires that we take a long view of life. The nitty-gritty dirt of our existence contains substance for wellness if we abide where we are planted. Look at the bamboo and see how it celebrates.

One particular type of bamboo puts down roots in thickets and jungles around the world. Throughout its life it perseveres toward a spectacular moment of realization. After decades of soil-searching and maturation, it magically and mysteriously opens its soul skyward. Inevitably, every 50 years or so, giant blades of grass trumpet their joy *together*.

All at once, simultaneously as a worldwide community, they burst into bloom in a unified anthem of glory. High in the sky, they proclaim a seed-scattering party, a jubilee. Wherever that species is to be found, whether in China, Japan, Korea, South America, North America or other distant places, stalks of bamboo burst into bloom all at once in a strong, vibrant expression of new life.

In the same way, we live now in the space of anticipatory joy. For persons of faith, authentic happiness is inevitable, relentless in its coming. This is because we are not alone.

THE HOMEWARD WHISTLE

Last week my cell phone chirped and a picture of my Mom lit up the screen as I pulled it from my shirt pocket. My sister Sue's text-messaged caption read: "Our beautiful mother! She seems to be a little better this morning. She tried whistling!"

Instantly I have flashbacks to another time: Mom standing on the porch steps, calling her children home to supper. Mom punctuated her summons with a piercing whistle.

~~~~~~~~~

We're all "home" now. Today as I write, I sit with my siblings at Mom's bedside in her Adult Family Home. Death is near. Figaro, a black and white cat known for his focused attendance upon dying residents is curled on Mom's lap. My sister Deanne is singing. During a lull, Agnes, a bright-eyed 101 year old resident comes in and asks, "Is she still with us. Is she gone?" She peers at Mom's face, leans down and says, "You're making a habit of sleeping, Betty. Get a stick on it. You know you need to get on with it or I'll bop you one. You know it's party time!" She smiles cheerfully, an encourager to all of us who watch Mom tarry on the cusp of death.

It has been a long journey. For Mom, it is now almost over. Along the way, she and Dad taught us the meaning and power of faith, hope and love. Sometimes with words, but more often than not, with unspoken grace.

In these hours of waiting, I am keenly aware that my parents have awakened hope within my heart. Through the years of my childhood and beyond, I've seen enough of the Holy to know that God is real. God has appeared time and again to me in places of despair. I've seen God shining through the faces of dying patients. And now I am seeing it in the restful countenance of my dying mother. What I've witnessed makes me yearn everyday for the healing that transcends medicinal cures.

But, until our world is healed of its brokenness, I'll keep returning to the storm-battered bamboo grove, trusting that the undergirding of God's root system of love will hold me and my siblings for however long we must wait and watch.

I will tarry in the grove, dig in the dirt, and devour the tender shoots of divine grace. Here in this place, I tune my heart to hear the Divine Parent whistling to me, calling me to partake of an infinite stream of resources. Unending grace. Unending love. Perfect healing for my broken spirit.

~~~~~~~~~

Mom died at 2 o'clock on a Friday morning in the springtime. I miss my Mother, just as I miss my Dad. In just a couple of days, my brothers, sisters, and I will gather to celebrate her journey. Then, not long after, I will return to the cauldron of traumas, codes and medical crises in my hospital.

What I have written in this book is deeply personal. I have lived and written what I know. In my case, the personal and professional dimensions of life intersect. And this life goes on and on and on. By now you know that spiritual caregiving is more than a profession. It becomes the life we live, a life that both exhausts and energizes. I hope that by now you have also encountered the Sacred herein in ways that equip you to navigate securely even when your world is shaking.

Blessings and peace!

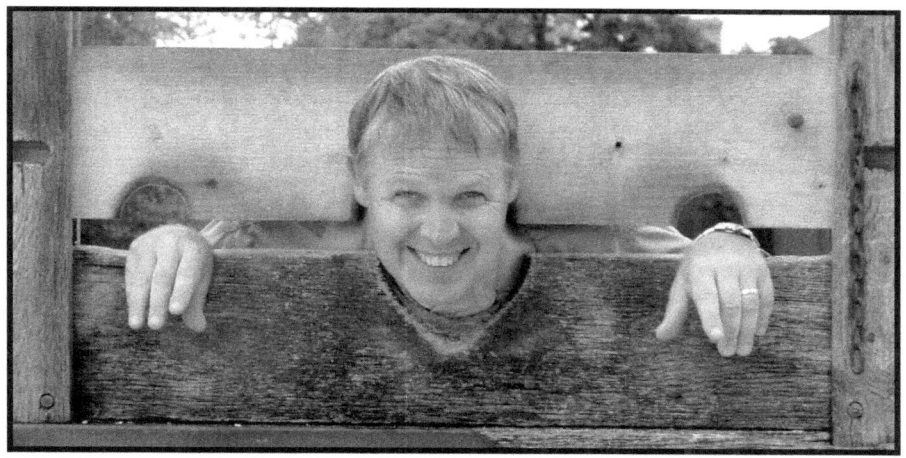

Tom Becraft is a Board Certified Chaplain and an award-winning author in the healthcare field. His booklet, *Crossing the Bridge: A Guide to End of Life Issues*, received the coveted 2011 Award for Spirituality and Diversity from Planetree, a patient-centered consortium of 600 hospitals in North America, South America, Asia, Europe and Australia.

Becraft currently serves as Lead Chaplain at Kadlec Regional Medical Center (KRMC), a 270-bed Level II Trauma hospital in Richland, WA. Concurrent with the award for *Crossing the Bridge*, KRMC became one of just sixteen Designated Planetree Patient-Centered Hospitals around the world, distinguishing itself for its advanced work in attending to the whole person.

Before transitioning into healthcare chaplaincy in 2005, Becraft served as a bilingual campus chaplain, college and high school educator and ordained minister at schools and churches in Japan, Hawaii and America's Northwest. He became a Board Certified Chaplain in the Association of Professional Chaplains in 2008. Each day he translates over three decades of cross-cultural ministry into attentiveness toward the needs, wishes and choices of patients, families and hospital staff, companioning with them on a quest for release from the shackles of emotional and spiritual pain.

He is inspired daily by his wife, Bonnie Oneonta-Becraft, a fellow Board Certified Chaplain who experienced a life-changing spinal cord injury in 1980 as the result of a surgical mishap. (This was followed by five months of hospitalization and subsequent rehabilitation to relearn all activities of daily living.) Tom and Bonnie are employed by Tri-Cities Chaplaincy (also known as The Chaplaincy), a nationally unique interfaith agency that provides in-home palliative care, hospice care, bereavement support, chaplaincy training, medical family therapy, and professional spiritual care services at multiple sites, including KRMC, in Washington State's Columbia Basin area. Tom was assigned to KRMC in 2006 to work fulltime with a team of dedicated colleagues.

Though the writing is Tom's, Bonnie's input is on every page of *A Bamboo Grove for the Soul*, especially in Chapter 4 where certain self-care contemplative practices are introduced. The scripts found within this fourth section were written by Tom and Bonnie together and provide opportunity for readers' personal creativity.

Tom has a master's degree (1980) in religion from Andrews University with a concentration in inter-religious, cross-cultural studies, and additional graduate work in education and counseling. His undergraduate degree was in theology with a minor in journalism (1974). While living in Japan he wrote two books in Japanese, one of which became a continuing education text for Japanese clergy. *A Bamboo Grove for the Soul* is Tom's first full-length book in English.

Bonnie has a master's degree in Marriage and Family Therapy from George Fox University (1999) and earlier undergraduate degrees in nursing (1972) and pastoral counseling (1992). As her health permits, she provides counseling support for individuals and family members whose relational dynamics have been disrupted by a catastrophic or chronic medical condition. Additionally, she provides post-graduate supervision and learning opportunities for persons seeking licensure in Washington and Oregon as Social Workers, Marriage and Family Therapists, or Mental Health Counselors. Like Tom, Bonnie is a minister, endorsed by Adventist Chaplaincy Ministries for healthcare chaplaincy.

The Becrafts live in Kennewick, WA where rivers, children and grandchildren converge with the seasons. Becrafts have a combined family of six adult children, their spouses, three grandchildren, and a "bucket list" of places to go, people to see, and experiences to share.

For additional spiritual care resources
go to the author's website: *www.Tom-Becraft.com*